The
HELPING PROFESSIONS
A CAREERS SOURCEBOOK

William R. Burger

Kingsborough Community College

Merrill Youkeles

Professor Emeritus at Kingsborough Community College

with

Fred B. Malamet
Franceska Blake Smith
Charles Guigno

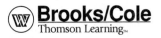

Brooks/Cole
Thomson Learning™

Australia • Canada • Denmark • Japan • Mexico • New Zealand • Philippines
Puerto Rico • Singapore • South Africa • Spain • United Kingdom • United States

Senior Editor: Lisa Gebo
Assistant Editor: Susan Wilson
Editorial Assistant: JoAnne von Zastrow
Production Editor: Howard Severson
Print Buyer: Stacey Weinberger
Text Designer: Adriane Bosworth

Copy Editor: Laura Larson
Cover Designer: Yvo Rezebos
Cover Images: PhotoDisc, Inc.
Compositor: Alphatype
Printer/Binder: West

Printed in the United States of America

2 3 4 5 6 03 02 01 00

For permission to use material from this text, contact us by
   web: www.thomsonrights.com
   fax: 1-800-730-2215
   phone: 1-800-730-2214

Wadsworth/Thomson Learning
10 Davis Drive
Belmont, CA 94002-3098
USA
www.wadsworth.com

International Headquarters
Thomson Learning
290 Harbor Drive, 2nd Floor
Stamford, CT 06902-7477
USA

UK/Europe/Middle East
Thomson Learning
Berkshire House
168-173 High Holborn
London WC1V 7AA
United Kingdom

Asia
Thomson Learning
60 Albert Street #15-01
Albert Complex
Singapore 189969

Canada
Nelson/Thomson Learning
1120 Birchmount Road
Scarborough, Ontario M1K 5G4
Canada

**Library of Congress
Cataloging-in-Publication Data**
Burger, William, 1949–
  The helping professions : a career sourcebook / William R. Burger, Marril Youkeles.
    p.   cm.
  Includes bibliographical references and index.
  ISBN 0-534-36475-6 (pbk.)
    1. Human services—Vocational guidance..
  2. Social service—Vocational guidance.
  3. Counseling—Vocational guidance.
  4. Mental health services—Vocational guidance. 5. Occupational therapy—Vocational guidance. I. Youkeles, Merrill. II. Title.
HV10.5.B85 1999
361'.0023'73—dc21   99-30488

 This book is printed on acid-free recycled paper.

Contents

Chapter 3

Careers as a Generalist Worker   29

Chapter 4

Careers in Social Work   39

Chapter 5

Careers in Counseling   52

Chapter 6

Careers in Psychology   73

Chapter 9

Careers in Art Therapy   119

Chapter 10

Careers in Dance/Movement Therapy   132

Chapter 11

Careers in Music Therapy   145

Index   158

Preface

The sourcebook is designed to provide career information not found in most human service texts. Therefore, it serves as a valuable complement to the existing textbooks in the field. It also serves as a resource for those who have yet to decide on a career path.

Hundreds of occupations involve helping people. Most of the professions described later offer several specialties that are important, interesting, and needed. Many of them will be only identified rather than described because of space limitations.

The human services professions focus on helping people who are having problems that prevent their functioning at a satisfactory level. These individuals may be hampered by emotional, cognitive, physical, or social problems, among others. This volume describes nine major professions in the human services field. They vary a great deal regarding the amount and type of training required for meeting sound professional standards. Because not all readers may be willing or able to seek extended higher education, it is fortunate that these helping professions permit a variety of career paths, with education and training ranging from high school to the doctoral level.

Why this book? Certainly others are available that describe human services careers. This book, however, does the following:

1. Identifies various settings of human services activities
2. Describes, through vignettes, the actual work activities of a typical human service worker in each of the fields.
3. Provides a realistic picture of some of the challenges and problems of each profession
4. Gives an idea of the salary levels and duties at various levels of training
5. Uses the experiences of professionals who not only have wide personal knowledge of the field but are also skilled at training human services workers
6. Provides information about educational licensing, certification, and steps needed to become a human services professional

How to Use the Book

The best way to use this book is to read it cover to cover. Even if you are certain that you want to be a recreation therapist, for example, the other career chapters contain valuable information for you. Like all human service workers, the recreation therapist usually works closely with psychologists, social workers, and other specialists. Specialists work in teams with generalists and other professionals. Therefore, you should know as much as possible about the skills, training, and point of view of the other professionals with whom you will be dealing. Your success as a human service worker often depends very much on your ability to work closely with coworkers and other professionals.

The first two chapters of this sourcebook provide essential background information regarding the field in general, the potential worker, and potential employers. Chapter 1 provides some idea of the scope of human services. Information about different types of agencies and their purposes and sponsorship is presented in addition to information regarding the consumers of human services. The effects of managed care on the provision of services will also be discussed, for they affect all human service professions in one way or another. In addition, the differences in descriptive and identifying terms within and between professions will become apparent.

Chapter 2 focuses on essential aspects involved in choosing a career. It discusses one's suitability to the field as well as what one looks for in a career. Furthermore, it provides information on what human service organizations look for in the potential worker. It highlights that choice of a career is a mutual choice of the worker and organization.

Chapter 3 through 11 describe specific careers. Each is first briefly defined and its features described. Reasons for choosing each career follow. Next is a brief account of the development of that profession. Some of the human services professions are old and well established. Others, however, are comparatively new and struggling to gain equal status and recognition with the more firmly rooted and familiar professions.

The bulk of each chapter is devoted to detailing the worker's duties and responsibilities and describing how you might become part of the profession. After providing an example of a day in the life of a worker in the field, we explore training, educational requirements, licensing, certification, and registration. The important matter of salary, with some representative job descriptions, is also covered.

Each career chapter includes an estimate of job availability in the future. This is, at best, an educated guess based on the best information at the time of writing. The job outlook depends on many factors that are difficult to predict, such as the level of government spending, which varies from year to year.

We suggest that you get the latest information about job availability after reading this book.

A long and unwieldy volume would be necessary to describe all of the human services careers. We selected the careers in this sourcebook based on several criteria. First, they have made significant contributions to the field of human services. Second, they illustrate the breadth and scope of human services careers. Third, they provide opportunities to use special skills and abilities needed to help people. Finally, because we recognize that not everyone is willing or able to pursue advanced education or training, we selected careers that demonstrate that it is possible to be a helpful and productive worker at different levels of training.

Because it is impossible to provide all available useful information of the careers included here, we do the next best thing. We add the professional organization for each career and cite references that are active in the field of human services. Many of them distribute career booklets and other aids. As you read about the field and gather information from other sources, it would be very helpful to set up a file on occupational information about each field that you are considering. Visiting agencies in the community that may have the kinds of jobs you are considering can also be very helpful. If you do plan to visit, call in advance to both obtain permission for the visit and to ensure that someone will have reserved time to talk with you.

Finally, many believe that computer literacy for those entering the field of human services is a skill that enhances one's chance in obtaining a desired position. Such a skill enables one to locate additional sources of employment possibilities and also provides the worker with a valuable tool to keep current with the changes in his or her profession.

Choosing a career in human services is a rewarding, exciting decision. We hope this book helps you explore the possibilities in your personal and professional journey.

ACKNOWLEDGMENTS

We wish to express our gratitude to the various individuals who provided advice and support, and for sharing their expertise with us during the preparation of this manuscript. In particular we must single out the contributions of Janice Strizever, Ellen Singer, Barbara Ladman, Sharon Allen, Brian Malamet, and Jennifer and Samuel Smith.

We continue to appreciate and value the efforts of our sponsoring editor, Lisa Gebo; our copy editor, Laura Larson; project editor, Howard Severson; and the entire production team for their diligence and support. Our thanks must also be given to the reviewers of this manuscript for their helpful suggestions and comments: Dr. Alan Kemp, Pierce College; Dr. Cynthia Poindexter, Boston University; Dr. Cris Robins, South Central Career College; Dr. Stephen Marson, University of North Carolina, Pembroke; and Prof. Charles Jaap, Pasco-Hernando Community College.

About the Contributors

Fred B. Malamet has been in the field of higher education for over 35 years as a teacher, counselor, and college administrator. He possesses a doctorate in administration and supervision of higher and adult education, a master's degree in guidance and student personnel administration, and a bachelor's degree in psychology. His interest in the field of human services has been lifelong and is something he has been able to include in his teaching as an associate professor in the Department of Behavioral Sciences at Kingsborough College of the City University of New York, along with his role as the dean of academic affairs. He considers curriculum development as one of the most important responsibilities, because the mission of the community college involves preparing graduates for careers in response to the trends and needs of society.

Franceska Blake Smith is an associate professor with the Department of Behavioral Sciences and Human Services at Kingsborough Community College of the City University of New York. She also directs Kingsborough's education associate program, which enrolls educators and support staff from New York City public schools. Fran earned a bachelor's degree from Harvard/ Radcliffe and master's and doctoral degrees from Columbia Teachers College, where she is an adjunct faculty member. Her research and teaching interests center on nontraditional and enthusiastic adult learners because she is (or aspires to be) such a learner herself.

Charles Guigno is a certified school psychologist. He received his doctorate degree in family and community education from Columbia University. For ten years, Charles worked as a private practitioner and private consultant for the New York City Board of Education and several nursing homes. He is currently on the faculty of the Mental Health and Human Services Program at Kingsborough Community College. He is particularly interested in family dynamics and alternate family lifestyles.

About the Authors

William R. Burger received his doctorate in social psychology, but his academic background also encompasses the fields of educational psychology and philosophy of education. While attending graduate school at Harvard University, he was awarded a research assistantship for his work in the area of community decision making. Bill is the former director of the Mental Health and Human Services Program and is currently chairperson of the Department of Behavioral Sciences and Human Services at Kingsborough Community College of the City University of New York. He has served as a consultant to a variety of human services programs in New York and Massachusetts, has lectured at various colleges and universities, and has written a number of guest editorial articles for various newspapers. Bill is coauthor, along with his colleague, Merrill Youkeles, of *Human Services in Contemporary America*, Fifth Edition.

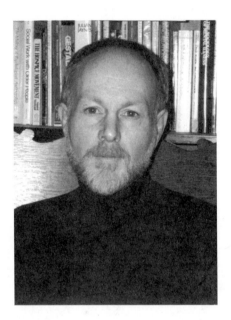

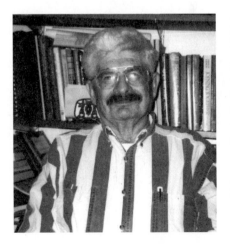

Merrill Youkeles, professor emeritus at Kingsborough Community College of the City University of New York, received his doctoral degree in studies on aging at Columbia University with the aid of a grant from the Administration on Aging. Merrill is a certified social worker who received his M.S.W. from the University of Pennsylvania and is the former director of the Mental Health and Human Services Program at Kingsborough College. He has more than 40 years of experience as a practitioner, consultant, and educator. His work in agencies, clinics, hospitals, and community organizations has given him a broad and realistic view of the human services field.

THE SCOPE OF
HUMAN SERVICES

Because the field of human services is so broad, it allows for almost limitless career opportunities in providing services to those in need. Confusion often occurs when one seeks to choose a specific career, among so many different possibilities, that will meet the needs of both the provider (student) and the consumer. Therefore, through offering general, but necessarily limited, information about the field of human services, we hope that you get some better idea of what it is that you are getting involved with. We sincerely urge you to explore your options further with knowledgeable career counselors, so that you can make a sound decision about the many possibilities for a career in the field of human services.

GENERAL FOCUS AND ROLES OF HUMAN SERVICE WORKERS

Human service workers deal with issues, problems, or concerns that affect people literally from the cradle to the grave. Some deal with abortion issues. Others relate to birth control, child care, child abuse, teenage pregnancy, teenage and adult violence and alcoholism, marriage, divorce, seniors' issues, and death.

On an institutional or societal basis, human service workers need to be concerned with hunger, violence, poverty, and racism, among other issues. Obviously, human service workers are unable to resolve all or any of these or other issues, but that point does not mean that they have no role to play. To the contrary, we strongly believe that the more complex and polarized our lives and society become, the greater the need will be for human service workers' support and expertise. Human service workers must become involved to some

1

degree with three major but general goals. These goals are closely interconnected and overlap one another regarding individual and institutional or societal issues. These three goals or purposes are:

- enhancing or improving the lives of individuals, groups, and society;
- preventing conditions that lead to the dysfunction of individuals,
  groups, and society; and
- helping individuals, groups, and society resolve existing problems that
  are causing dysfunction and prohibiting growth and desired change.

SPONSORSHIP OF AGENCIES/INSTITUTIONS

For human service workers to be able to provide needed services, they need
the support of the community. We wish to emphasize that the support of "the
community" refers to the support of generally more than one of the many enti-
ties that make up the community. It consists of foundations; businesses; religious, civic, philanthropic, governmental, social, and educational organizations,
among others, as well as concerned families and individuals. These groups
and individuals are the sponsors of institutions, agencies, and individuals that
provide the desired and needed services.

There are three major categories of sponsors and/or agencies or institutions that provide human services: (1) tax-supported or governmental agencies,
(2) private nonprofit agencies, and (3) profit-making institutions. In addition,
a significant number of human service workers enter into private practice,
which is in effect a profit-making endeavor.

A brief look at each of these groups will provide a clearer picture of how
they are interrelated. It might also help you in making decisions about with
whom and how you want to become involved in the human services.

Governmental or tax-supported human service agencies and programs are
developed and funded by elected governmental officials. They determine the
amount and kind of funding, as well as the overall policy of the institution. In
effect, the government—federal, state, or local—is the sponsor of the agency.
If, for example, enough individuals and groups in a town or county decide
that a senior center is desired or needed to meet the needs of their older adult
population, they ask their representatives to provide, through the town or
county budget, the required services. On local issues, the request is generally
more easily dealt with than the more complex and involved issues that usually
characterize state and federal problems.

Nongovernmental or private nonprofit institutions provide services that
governmental agencies do not or cannot provide or support. Private nonprofit
institutions are sponsored and supported by concerned individuals, groups,

and communities. The funding and overall policy of agencies such as family and adoption agencies, settlement houses, and hospitals, among many others, is determined by a board of directors. The members of these boards generally consist of prominent and/or affluent, concerned individuals in the community. They frequently come from many different backgrounds, which often include business, health, religion, education, politics, philanthropy, or residents in the community where the service is provided. These individuals and groups raise money from foundations, individuals, and businesses, among other sources. The institutions they support are not permitted to make a profit. If the income from the services is more than the cost of services, those monies are put back into the institution to pay off debts or to purchase new equipment or services. Various governmental agencies are responsible to make sure that these private nonprofit institutions maintain a nonprofit status through the proper use of funds, the provision of appropriate services, and other criteria.

Private profit-making agencies and private practitioners need the support of individuals, groups, and the community. Very rarely are these institutions and practitioners completely independent. As do the nonprofit institutions, the profit-making institutions are, if they are professional, involved with licensing and certification of their services and personnel. Professional organizations also are important to these institutions and individuals. On a very practical basis, if individuals in the community choose not to buy or pay for the offered services, the private agencies and practitioners will fall by the wayside. Local community and other groups, in addition, often are determining factors in whether a group home or psychiatric clinic can be located in their community.

Profit-making agencies do provide services that the nonprofit sector does not or cannot offer. They also serve populations that are often not eligible for services provided by the nonprofit agencies. Many of these organizations are also run or controlled by a board of directors. The major purpose of these boards is to assure that a sufficient profit is made to provide an adequate income for those providing the services. These institutions and practitioners are a significant part of the human service field.

MANAGED CARE

A brief discussion of managed care is warranted, for its introduction and rapid growth have had a tremendous impact on a very significant number of human service providers. Managed care, a method of providing primary health services, was devised to achieve at least three goals:

1. To contain and retard the rapid increases in the cost of providing health and medical services by governmental, nonprofit, and profit-making health organizations
2. To maintain a reasonable and manageable level of cost to individuals, groups, and business subscribers who purchase health insurance
3. To assure the profitability of the insurance companies that sell and provide health insurance policies

These goals are reached primarily through decisions made by persons other than the direct provider determining the need for treatment, the timing, and the type and length of the treatment or service. Anyone seeking a career in the human services should explore this area thoroughly and carefully, because it affects most, if not all, human service professions and professionals.

TYPES OF AGENCIES/INSTITUTIONS

In this section we will identify many different types of agencies in which human service workers are employed, including tax-supported governmental agencies, private nonprofit institutions, and private profit-making services. This discussion can help you determine to some degree what specific career or specialty you wish to pursue. Many of these institutions provide services and deal with issues requiring several different professional disciplines. For this reason, and others, we repeat our caution and urging that you investigate and research, personally, each agency that you might consider for employment. This effort on your part will help you make a knowledgeable and sound decision regarding your career.

Nationwide agencies include the Red Cross, Salvation Army, Armed Services hospitals and clinics, federal prisons, justice systems, and federal welfare agencies, among others.

Statewide and local agencies include hospitals, family agencies, adoption, child care and child protection agencies, senior centers, nursing homes, home care, shelters, and meals-on-wheels. In addition, there are agencies that offer services to teenage mothers, teen gangs, single parents, and job and parental training. Agencies helping those living in poverty include welfare programs such as food stamps, job training, housing and shelter programs, as well as medical help. Also included are school and after-school programs, settlement houses, YMCAs, and other recreation and socialization programs. Rehabilitation programs are available for the physically disabled, emotionally disabled, learning disabled, drug addicts, and alcoholics. The justice system has its parole and probation programs in aiding juvenile and adult prisoners. Various religious groups provide counseling and services around illness and death.

These and many other kinds of agencies offer so many more programs and services that provide employment opportunities on so many different professional levels. The people whom they help will be discussed in the next section.

Whom Do You Help?

You should realize by now that human service workers help a tremendous range of people whose situations and problems match their variety and possibly their number.

On entering a helping profession, you might work with the elderly, juvenile delinquents, prisoners, poor people, wealthy people, retarded children, drug addicts, or even healthy people who are not seriously disturbed. Each group has its own special problems and challenges. We will try to give you a feel for what it would be like to work with a few groups so you can begin to think about what kind of people you would prefer to work with and why you feel the way you do.

To avoid some confusion, however, it is necessary at this point for you to become aware of the many different descriptive and identifying terms that may mean the same thing and be used interchangeably. For example the terms *patient, consumer,* or *client* often refers to the same individual. One might prefer calling a seventy-five-year-old person *older adult, senior citizen, aged, elderly,* or some other descriptive term. Different professions and professionals have different preferences based on their perception of which terms are more accurate, more dignified, less condescending, or more politically correct. We use the different terms in this book to help you become aware of some of these differences.

The Elderly

By the year 2030, the elderly will probably make up 20 percent of the population. This sharp increase in the number of elderly will have a great impact on helping services because the chances of needing help increase with age. The increased life span of people today brings with it pleasures and problems. Problems resulting from enforced retirement, limited income, loss of status, or a growing sense of hopelessness often accompany old age. These issues have become a major concern because of the growing number of older people. Workers in the senior centers attempt to help older adults remain as independent and as happy as possible in their last years. Social workers, psychiatrists, psychologists, recreation therapists, and generalist human service workers make up the staff of the centers and other agencies serving older adults.

The decline in physical vitality of older persons is often accompanied by emotional difficulties. For example, the elderly frequently face the loss of friends and loved ones and feel less useful to others than before. Retirement from the workforce typically means reduced income and loss of the support group associated with the work setting. There is a growing awareness that we need to provide more preventive services for senior citizens. Special agencies such as YMCAs, settlement houses, and senior citizen centers are offering programs for the elderly. Social workers, recreational therapists, and generalists are all involved in this effort to prevent the older person from becoming depressed and lonely. Home visits, free transportation, escort services, financial advice, and recreational activities are just some of the services provided.

The elderly person who cannot live independently may be placed in a senior residence, a nursing home, a hospital for chronic diseases, or a mental hospital, depending on the kind or care required. Those confined to mental hospitals may suffer from senility, brain damage, or severe depression. Some of the places where we care for our elderly admittedly have a depressing atmosphere. However, working with the elderly can be very satisfying in settings with active therapeutic and recreational programs.

A major type of nonmedical, nonresidential facility serving the older adult is the senior or multiservice center. At first these were places for older adults to meet and enjoy themselves. Today there are over 5,000 centers serving the varied needs of older adults.

The Poor

Although the United States is one of the wealthiest nations on earth, many Americans are not sharing in the general affluence. Reports indicate that thousands of Americans are going hungry. Many live in poverty. According to the poverty line established by the Social Security Administration, in a recent year over 15 percent of the population were living in poverty.

These poor Americans include unemployed workers, elderly persons on fixed incomes, farm workers displaced by new machinery, persons who lack saleable job skills, and others. Minority group members, recent immigrants, and women are disproportionately represented among the ranks of the poor.

Within poor communities one finds a series of interconnected problems. Unemployment, welfare dependency, alcoholism, drug addiction, disease, crime, and mental illness all seem to feed on one another. The hopelessness of chronic poverty sometimes leads to a lifestyle based on living for immediate pleasures. The slum neighborhoods of our large cities can yield mental patients, criminals, and juvenile delinquents.

Helping professionals from middle-class backgrounds are often puzzled by the self-defeating behaviors of some poor people. Rather than tackle problems head-on, some poor persons may try to escape them by means of alcohol or drugs. Their life experiences have drained many of them of any hope for a better future.

Experienced workers know that the poor person may try to manipulate the worker for the sake of some immediate gain. When the worker encourages the client to consider a more constructive lifestyle, it becomes obvious that beginning a new way of life is a challenging and frightening undertaking. When a poor person leaves the institution where he or she has been confined and returns to the old neighborhood, all of the pressures that helped create the problem in the first place must be faced again.

Settlement houses, YMCAs, community development programs, and similar agencies are shifting their efforts to helping people ease the physical and emotional impact of poverty and to deal with family and interpersonal problems. In addition, they provide recreation, cultural educational programs, and information and referrals. Community development programs were established to meet the needs of unserved to underserved communities. These agencies are staffed by social workers, psychologists, psychiatrists, vocational and rehabilitation counselors, and generalist human service workers.

Good intentions do not always lead to success in working with poor people. This is not said to discourage the potential helper but to point out that we have not yet developed sure-fire techniques to solve great social problems. Part of the excitement for the worker lies in the effort to develop individual programs and approaches that will have an impact on poor people. These kinds of approaches can only grow out of a sophisticated understanding of the situation facing the poor person in America today.

Juvenile Delinquents

The elderly and the dependent poor in the United States are often not considered fully responsible or productive persons. To some extent, teenagers are in a similar position. Neither adults nor children, they lack a clear sense of identity. Their in-between status probably contributes to the rebellious and defiant behavior that some exhibit.

Few people are aware of the magnitude of today's juvenile delinquency problem. Although boys are responsible for most juvenile crimes, the rate for girls has gone up sharply in recent years. Criminal activity among youngsters is by no means confined to the inner cities. Similar high rates have been reported for youngsters from suburban and rural areas.

What kind of background produces a child who engages in destructive criminal activity? Delinquent youths are likely to come from broken homes and, in particular, from homes disrupted by divorce rather than from the death of a parent. A pattern of rejection by one or both parents is often found, along with inconsistent discipline by the parents. Frequently, the parents of delinquents alternate harsh, brutal punishment with periods of neglect or disinterest. The child lacks respect for his or her parents and later shows a similar attitude toward teachers, police, and other authority figures. The youngster grows up hostile, defiant, and full of aggressive urges toward others.

Some juveniles become part of a regular, organized gang. In most juvenile gangs, the members share a sense of loyalty for each other but feel rejected and unwanted by the larger society. This rejection has some basis in fact. Most gang members lack either the ability or motivation to do well in school. They drop out at the earliest possible age, usually sixteen, and then quickly learn that they qualify for very few jobs. And the jobs that are available are low paying with few chances for advancement. It seems like there is no place for the teenager in the outside world. Within the gang, such youths might feel that they can experience a sense of acceptance not possible elsewhere.

Some juvenile offenders, particularly those who commit violent crimes, may eventually be sent to a training school or "reformatory," as such places were once called. In the best of such institutions, the youth receives psychological counseling in addition to educational and occupational training. Hopefully, the offender may then return home with a good chance of fitting into society. Unfortunately, most training schools are understaffed and overcrowded. Usually the buildings of the school are outdated and inadequate. It is not surprising, then, that the rate of recidivism (repeating the same criminal behavior) is very high for delinquents sent to such schools. There are, of course, some excellent schools and programs that do a good job of genuinely "reforming" the offender, and these can be very rewarding and challenging places to work for helping professionals.

Some experts believe large-scale preventive programs are needed. Such programs should provide a wide range of educational, occupational, and social opportunities for teenagers. One goal would be to involve the community as much as possible in working with the juvenile, who often feels that nobody really cares. Specific programs might include employment training, group counseling, and life skills training.

Criminals

The crime rate, although dropping significantly recently, is higher in the United States than in most other industrialized nations. In 1998, the FBI reported that 12.5 million serious crimes were committed in the United States, including homicide, rape, robbery, aggravated assault, and auto theft. This figure included only crimes that were reported to law enforcement agencies; the actual rate is undoubtedly higher.

A small percentage of crimes are committed by so-called psychopathic personalities. They may be found in the ranks of businesspeople, lawyers, politicians, doctors, and evangelists as well as among drug dealers and prostitutes. Psychopaths are typically intelligent and often come across as charming to their victims. Essentially, they do not feel strong guilt or anxiety. The lack of guilt combined with apparent sincerity enable psychopaths to successfully con other people. They are not the sort of people who come to community clinics seeking help. They come into contact with helping professionals only when caught in the machinery of the criminal justice system.

Not all criminals are psychopaths. Most professional criminals, including drug dealers, burglars, and forgers, are motivated mainly by a desire for easy money. Unlike the psychopath, they form close relationships with others and may feel a strong sense of loyalty to a criminal group. Many criminals were raised in homes in which hostility toward the larger culture was the rule. As he or she matures, the typical criminal specializes in a particular kind of crime and develops a characteristic method of operation. The burglar or forger usually does not commit crimes of violence. Unlike true psychopaths, most professional criminals have good control of their impulses and are able to profit from experience. The real professional accepts the hazards of the criminal lifestyle and usually adapts well to prison routine.

Presently, more than 1,700,000 persons are serving in federal, state, and local prisons, with an additional one million released on probation. These offenders are predominantly the "losers" of our society: the poor, the disadvantaged, and many minority group members. The rich and powerful are often able to evade punishment for offenses that would send a poor person to jail.

Our correctional facilities fail to protect the public as criminals are constantly being recycled back into the community where they are likely to repeat the same crime. This cycle is not surprising because our prisons are not well designed to help an offender learn how to function productively in a free society. In most prisons the regimentation is so severe that the inmate loses any sense of individuality or responsibility. The prisoner spends time exclusively with other criminals, and antisocial attitudes usually harden. Relatively little effort is devoted to treatment, rehabilitation, or job training.

The many inadequacies of our criminal justice system have discouraged persons in the helping professions from considering jobs in this area. Only a tiny percentage of persons working in penal institutions are involved in treatment. The rest are guards, administrators, and support personnel. Only a minority of correctional personnel work with the critical areas of probation and parole. Again, the quality and quantity of such supervision is open to serious question. There is some basis for the hope that corrections will be more attractive to helping personnel in the near future. Several kinds of model or "therapeutic" prisons are currently being studied. In addition, studies are going forward on new approaches to parole and probation that may serve as models for future efforts.

At present, the best opportunities for treatment within the criminal justice system are in probation. The probation officer has a chance to work with offenders on a one-to-one basis and also has the option of establishing group therapy programs. Many probation officers feel they could be more effective if they were not given huge caseloads. This is another way in which government practices false economy. Probation officers can be successful only if caseloads are reasonable and programs well designed.

For both juvenile and adult criminals, additional services are available. These are court and corrections services that help individuals and families involved in judicial or legal proceedings. In criminal cases, probation and parole services might include personal counseling, referrals, or rehabilitation counseling. In other cases involving juveniles and family courts, testing, information, and consulting services are provided by various mental health personnel. Civil cases, such as adoption, support, and conciliation proceedings, are provided with consultation, information, referral, and guidance services. As in most other settings, psychiatrists, social workers, psychologists, and vocational and rehabilitation counselors are the type of personnel hired to provide these necessary services.

The Mentally Challenged

The mentally challenged have been referred to as the "mentally retarded" or "mentally handicapped." The word *challenged* is certainly a more encouraging designation. The mentally challenged differ from the other groups we have discussed in one critical respect: their disability results from subnormal intelligence.

One aspect of intelligence is how quickly a person is able to learn new material. The first intelligence tests were designed to identify children who could not be expected to keep up with a normal class. The persons we call challenged are those who score well below the average of 100 on intelligence tests. To be more exact, individuals with IQs below 70 are usually classified as mentally challenged.

The number of mentally challenged people in the United States is about six million, a very significant portion of population. The mentally challenged group is subdivided into four smaller groups: the mildly, moderately, severely, and profoundly challenged.

The majority of mentally challenged persons are in the mild category. The mildly mentally challenged person may not stand out as obviously challenged.

This person can learn practical self-care skills and master reading and arithmetic at a grade school level. As an adult, he or she can usually work but might need occasional guidance and support.

The person who is moderately mentally challenged is often poorly coordinated but can eventually learn to communicate with others on a simple level. He or she can master some basic health and safety habits but makes little progress in reading or arithmetic. The moderately mentally challenged person can usually travel alone in familiar places but is not capable of living alone. Most persons in this category are able to work in sheltered conditions.

The severely mentally challenged person does not develop communication skills beyond a few simple words. He or she may be able to learn self-feeding and other forms of self-care but will always require supervision in a protected environment. There is greater likelihood that the individual will show a physical defect or deformity. The severely mentally challenged person is usually, but not always, capable of walking and getting around.

The profoundly mentally challenged person shows retarded development in all areas of functioning. Speech remains primitive, and there is little ability to master self-care skills. This person requires nursing care but may be able to learn some basic use of the legs, hands, and jaw. He or she is often institutionalized and can be maintained in the home only with heroic effort.

It is well known that a person's surroundings during the early years of life can have a lasting effect on intelligence. For example, children who are raised in uninteresting settings such as some orphanages, hospitals, and institutions tend to have lower IQs than those raised in stimulating, complex settings. The amount of parental warmth, touching, and cuddling also affects both personality and intelligence. Children raised in poverty conditions tend to score lower than average on intelligence tests. This fact is the center of an intense controversy, with some experts maintaining that the lowered scores result from a deprived background and others saying that inheritance plays a role here. However, no one would deny that early training has an important effect on intelligence.

The fact that mentally challenged people cannot be expected to function at a normal level does not mean that they cannot improve. In fact, many can learn to improve their skills very significantly. Of course, the degree of change that can be expected is related to the level of the IQ. Those in the mildly challenged range have the potential to show the most improvement, and these comprise the majority of cases. Most mentally challenged persons do not need to be institutionalized and can be helped by educational and training schools in the community. Classes for the mildly challenged that teach reading, occupational skills, and budgeting have been very successful in helping the students become independent and useful members of society. Classes for the moderately challenged emphasize self-care and other basic skills needed to get along in the world. In many cases, simple job skills can also be learned.

Unfortunately, many feel that education and training programs for the mentally challenged are not doing an adequate job. Overcrowding, insufficient funding, and inadequate staffing are just some of the problems that plague these special schools. Millions of mentally challenged persons could become self-supporting if they received the right kind of occupational training. Their potential contribution is being wasted because of the absence of proper training. Despite some improvement in recent years, the majority of the mentally challenged still do not receive the level of services they need. One exception are mentally challenged persons whose families can afford to send them to one of the many excellent private facilities that are available. These private schools are generally beyond the financial reach of the average working-class family, however.

CONCLUSION

As you read this chapter, you may have been surprised by the great variety of people who receive human services of one kind or another. In addition to those described here, human service workers attempt to support or help many others, including the victims of violence, people with physical disabilities, the emotionally ill, the homeless, the victims of natural disasters, and dysfunctional families, among several others. Human service workers tend to specialize in one kind of client or patient. Working with the mentally challenged is very different from working with alcoholics, which in turn is different than dealing with drug addicts. Many workers have strong feelings about the kind of population with which they want to work. Some do not want to work with mentally challenged clients, whereas others would prefer working with them. Some workers have a special flair for working with youth gangs; others would refuse to do so. The point is that in such a diverse field, it is OK to have these sorts of preferences. Hopefully, the human service worker should have an understanding of his or her feelings about different groups of people and feel comfortable about personal choices.

The following chapters will provide you with many other examples of who needs help, who helps them, and where the help is provided.

ARE YOU SUITED FOR THE FIELD?

While you are considering a career in human services, think about how you might be suited for one of the jobs in this varied field. Look at your personal assets and liabilities before investing. Put into different terms, consider your personal characteristics, motivations, likes and dislikes, and beliefs that would help you in your chosen career rather than become obstacles for you to overcome. Are you a person who already possesses many of the qualities that would contribute toward becoming an effective professional helper? Take a good look at yourself and begin to consider certain areas relevant to your career selection. As in any profession, skills must be developed and a variety of additional knowledge must be obtained.

In most important decisions, we have to make a judgment about what is best for ourselves. We generally attempt to clarify our thoughts by breaking down the larger decision into smaller parts and examining each part in relation to the larger decision. We will follow a similar process in this chapter by approaching the larger decision of a career choice in the helping professions and exploring each segment of that choice.

This chapter explores reasons, expectations, and motivations for choosing a career in this field. Because there is no one "right" reason behind a career choice, we will discuss a variety of possible reasons. This includes your self-concept, which is essentially the way in which you view yourself. Do you like or dislike yourself? What contributes to your likes or dislikes? Do you see yourself solely as a student, housewife, teacher, or parent? We also discuss what human service organizations look for in their selection of new staff.

The basic tool of helping professionals is themselves; thus, we must learn to recognize and understand how to best use our personal qualities. This, of course, demands sufficient self-knowledge and self-awareness before you can hope to fully develop various aspects of your personality. To help you become more aware of yourself, we will explore the various types of relationships experienced by human beings. An appropriate beginning would consider the most basic element common to all the areas within the helping profession—people.

RELATIONSHIPS

People need people for a variety of reasons and need each other in a number of ways. The ability to establish and maintain different types of relationships with people is indeed an integral part of life as well as within the helping professions.

Business Relationships

Various relationships can be found in work environments. You might be a stockbroker working within a firm with other brokers and clients. You might be an electrician working in a shop with other electricians. You might be a sales clerk working within a large department store with other salespeople and a wide range of customers. Whatever your place and type of work, your main purpose in being there is to perform your job effectively, but the quality of your relationships with your coworkers may be a key to performing your job well.

The most common example of a business relationship is the seller-buyer. These relationships may be formal with rules and regulations that govern interaction between people. Such posted signs as "Don't talk to the bus driver while the bus is in motion" and "No customers allowed in work area" are examples. An automotive mechanic attempting to fix your car, a laundry person cleaning your clothes, or a painter preparing your house for its annual paint job are relationships in which you, as the consumer of a service, are paying another person solely for his or her abilities and expertise. Hopefully you trust their competence in performing the job correctly, but it is not essential in this relationship that you particularly like them or feel loving and trusting toward them as people. Neither do you need to share the details of your life with them.

Personal Relationships

These relationships include friends, family, and loved ones and are more informal and spontaneous than business relationships. A friendship is formed because you value the qualities of the other person. You may like this person's sense of humor or share the same interests, and you trust each other. There is a greater degree of intimacy within this alliance because you are free to choose your friends.

A family relationship consists of connections acquired through birth. In this form of relationship, people tend to share common experiences, which usually—but not always—promotes caring and understanding of one another. Because you are born into a specific group of people we call "family," it does not automatically mean you love, care for, or enjoy the other people within your family. The family relationship usually calls for a certain amount of cooperation and interdependence if it is to function effectively. Often this effectiveness is hampered by competition among brothers and sisters and resentment from the children toward the parents and vice versa.

Love relationships are another form of personal relationships. Love, like other intense emotional feelings, is a somewhat stronger connection between people. Because it is a stronger feeling than liking, it suggests a greater need and attraction for the other person. Love is not limited to certain aspects of the person. You may love a specific thing about a person, or you may love the way a person makes you feel. Often a love relationship would include a physical connection as well, as in the case of lovers, and husbands and wives. It is possible to love certain aspects of a person and to dislike other aspects. Although love suggests this strong feeling for the other, it does not always mean there is respect or sharing within the relationship.

Competitive Relationships

This form of relationship may be found in various aspects of life, especially within sports; for example, a tennis player pits his or her knowledge, abilities, and training against another. Clearly the goal of this sort of relationship is to beat the other person at a specific game or contest and emerge the winner. It is not important that you care for, trust, or like your opponent. What is important is your ability to outmaneuver that person. In the case of team competition, it is important for you to cooperate with your teammates and depend on them to perform their assignments well.

Professional Relationships

These are closely related to the business type but different. As in business relationships, professional relationships also tend to be formal, with rules and regulations governing the quality of interaction and tending to remove spontaneity and informality. Examples include a lawyer and client, physician and patient, and teacher and student. As the dictionary definitions suggest, "a professional is someone characterized as conforming to the technical or ethical standards of a profession." Professional people are those who usually acquire a high degree of formal education, training, and skills. This formal training requires the ability to conform to certain codes of conduct. These codes of conduct are usually enforced by societal laws. Lawyers, teachers, and medical doctors must take certain examinations demonstrating their knowledge of these codes. In certain instances, as with medical doctors, they must even take an oath pledging their conformity to these rules.

Because of these parameters, the relationships that develop tend to be more structured and patterned. In your relationship with your lawyer, for example, it is not necessarily important that you share intimate details of your life or that you really like him or her as a person. You are paying a fee to the lawyer for professional ability in understanding and translating the law. As with teacher and student relationships, the teacher's ability to teach and motivate the student to learn is of sole importance.

The Helping Relationship

When problems develop within the various forms of relationships previously described, people may seek some form of help from another type of trained professional. This process of seeking help and the resultant relationship between the trained helper and his or her client form a new, unique form of relationship we call the *helping relationship*. This is a form of the professional relationship described earlier. Working in the helping professions requires an ability to form constructive, healthy, meaningful relationships with others. It develops such feelings as trust, respect, openness, caring, and sharing. The helper and the client enter into this relationship for the purpose of helping the client solve problems.

Although the helping relationship is an alliance between people, it is an unequal alliance. The efforts at helping are focused exclusively on the client. However, the helper also gains from the relationship in different ways. Human beings have a universal need to help others. Religious teachings have illustrated this need in the idea that "it is better to give than to receive." Within this helping process the helper is likely to experience a strengthened self-image, or feel better about him- or herself as a result of being asked to help someone.

As helpers, we must assume responsibility for creating an environment in which people feel comfortable enough to work toward reaching their desired goals. It must be understood that trying to help someone with the intention of changing them or molding them to conform to some standard of behavior can actually hinder the relationship. As a helper, you are there primarily to meet the client's needs, not for the client to meet your needs. Each of us in the field of human services has different reasons for being there. Your being aware of these reasons, as the helper, will enable you to understand more of what you are trying to accomplish from the helping process.

Another element common to most helping relationships is limited time. The helper and client form an alliance for the purpose of solving a specific problem. When the goal has been reached, the relationship is finished. It may last a single meeting or extend over a year or more. As a result of this time factor, another important element is the type of alliance, contract, or agreement made between the helper and client. A helper, because he or she must be aware of his or her own limitations, must not agree to help the client beyond these boundaries or else risks being unable to meet promises, thus facing further difficulty in the relationship.

The process of effectively helping someone has been referred to as both a science and an art. The science portion is made clear by the volumes of research involving human behavior. Patterns among people in various situations and universal human needs have become somewhat clear. The art portion is a little less clear. It refers to how helpers interpret the research evidence and use it individually within the helping process. This demands some degree of creativity, intuition, and a "feeling" for the other person. Just as in the world of painting, an artist may have received in-depth training in the various styles and techniques of painting, but when he or she sits alone with a canvas, it is creativity and feeling that usually distinguish a good painting from a great one.

A person needs help when personal abilities are not sufficient to overcome a difficulty. Normal functioning is usually hampered by one or more of the following areas:

1. A specific crisis that seems too large to overcome and overwhelms abilities to cope with it—for example, death of a loved one, an accident, or separation/divorce
2. Difficulty knowing the resources available to deal with the problem, such as where to go and what to do
3. Lack of desire to seek the necessary resources and becoming stuck and feeling that there is no way out
4. Insufficient skills to find the available information and, therefore, not knowing which alternatives to pursue

A major characteristic of the professional helping relationship is helping people grow. The person seeking help should be actively engaged in selecting the goals of personal growth. The desired help may take the form of a consultation requesting additional information, such as in drug rehabilitation centers, alcoholic treatment programs, or mental health clinics. Help in decision making and solving various problems such as choosing or changing a career, coping with relatives, feeling less anxious or depressed, or simply exploring the manner in which clients see themselves and the outside world encourages personal growth and satisfaction.

Problems in relationships and poor communication often occur when people fail to recognize some basic ideas. Several commonly accepted views contribute to the development of a healthy and constructive helping relationship:

- All people have problems at one time or another.
- Seeking help for problems is a sign of strength, not a sign of weakness.
- No one is all good or all bad.
- People's behavior does not always reveal their inner thoughts and feelings.
- All people are unique.
- All people have valid feelings.
- Do not expect or demand perfection from self or others.
- Understand the need for help.
- Know your own strengths, weaknesses, and limitations.
- All people have a need for security and dependence as well as for growth and independence.
- All people need to experience their lives as meaningful.
- Know how long help is needed.

As mentioned previously, helpers must possess an awareness of themselves and their needs. They must know how to satisfy these needs and understand how these needs affect their relationships. As one can see, becoming an effective helper is not just a matter of showing some degree of competence. It involves not only skills and training but knowledge of self. To develop this essential self-knowledge, we must look at the various ways we choose to define ourselves. The following section explores the factors that contribute to this understanding.

IMPORTANCE OF SELF-CONCEPT

As no two people are exactly alike, no two professional helpers use the same treatment. This diversity seems ever-present. No training, framework of theories, or experience will cover all situations. What, then, makes the difference between a good and a poor helper? Much of the current research in this field has focused on this question. Although the evidence is not overwhelmingly conclusive, it does point out that the helper's ability to use his or her own specific characteristics and attributes in such a manner as to establish an excellent helping relationship is critical. This concept of using oneself as a primary tool for helping is often referred to as the *conscious use of self*. The primary tool the helper must always depend on is him- or herself. To best use oneself in this manner, one must have sufficient self-knowledge. We will focus here on the development of this essential knowledge.

Our views of ourselves and the outside world seem so real and accurate to us that we seldom doubt our views about people and events. Our values and beliefs function as a yardstick by which we measure others. Because people behave in terms of their views and beliefs, effective helping should start with the helper's understanding of his or her own personal views and how all people form views of themselves. This involves understanding the overlapping terms *self* and *self-concept*.

The *self* is made up of what we consciously think about ourselves. Literally thousands of different aspects and ideas make up this image of self. When we use "I" and "me" in conversation, we are referring to this system of self. One of the unique things about human beings is our ability to step outside ourselves and ask, "What's important to me?" We will find these answers contained in the self.

The major development of the self occurs at birth when we interact with our environment. Significant people all around us give us views of ourselves. People may tell us we are kind, thoughtful, wise, nasty, selfish, or uncooperative. We may decide to accept some of these views and start to see ourselves in that manner. The self, therefore, contains all our values, beliefs, attitudes, and feelings. It is through the self that one's personality is expressed. It is the sum total of everything expressed as "me." The self has often been described as the inner world in which one lives.

The *self-concept* is how we feel about the various aspects of self. What aspects of self do we like or dislike? Obviously, self and self-concept are part of the same system. One part of the system defines your traits, whereas the other part determines how you feel about these characteristics. For example, a person might view himself as Bill Johnson—teacher, good husband and father, middle-aged, white male, and terrible dancer. These views and beliefs about himself make up the self-concept of Bill Johnson. It is clear that the self-concept does not stop with a description of self. It goes one step further and includes a qualitative judgment of each characteristic.

Professionals generally accept that if you want to become more effective as a helper, you must start with yourself. Our personalities are the basic tools we use within the helping relationship. We must be able to act immediately and spontaneously to situations that arise within the helping process. No matter how we may try to avoid it, helpers often become models of behavior to be imitated by the client. We must be highly aware of what values, beliefs, and attitudes we convey. It is only through self-examination that we can begin to understand what aspects of ourselves would be most beneficial to use within the helping process. The kind of self-awareness can be obtained by a desire and commitment to self-growth: a desire to know more about yourself and how you influence others. It is not uncommon for helpers to obtain counseling for themselves or participate in a wide variety of groups aimed at self-exploration.

The goals of professional helpers can be reached by entering into a relationship that includes this kind of give and take. The amount of giving, however, is possible only to the degree that the helpers feel fulfilled and good about themselves. For example, if a human services professional is physically ill, he or she cannot help others in the most effective way. Similarly, if the worker feels emotionally deprived, unsatisfied, and unfulfilled, the helping process becomes impaired. A person must have a sense of adequacy to form a healthy relationship and commit to helping others. Psychologists have referred to this idea as *positive self-regard* or *high self-esteem*. In short, only when you feel basically good about yourself can you go beyond your own needs and give attention to others. Whether you are old or young, fat or thin, of any race or physical ability, if you like yourself, you will usually relate well to others.

BELIEFS—MOTIVATION

The helper's value system is of special importance in working with people. Even though our beliefs comprise one aspect of the self-system, their influence on the helping process demands closer examination. The ways in which we behave as helpers will depend on our concepts and ideas about people. Actually, it does not matter whether the ideas we have about people are accurate or false; if we accept and believe them, they affect our behavior.

Consider the example of a professional marriage counselor. His beliefs will certainly have an effect on how he views and carries out his job responsibilities. Right now the marriage counselor is working with a couple who is considering a divorce as the solution to their problems. If he believes that every couple should stay together above all else, he might be biased in the direction of advising the couple to stay together. If, on the other hand, the counselor's beliefs are that the current state of marriage is nothing more than a piece of legal paper, and people unhappy with their relationship should leave it, his professional judgment and counseling may be biased in suggesting the couple separate.

Along with beliefs, a person's motivation and reasons for entering the field have an effect on his or her performance as a helper. It should be clearly understood that there is no one correct motivation for choosing this field. The personal reasons for helpers joining the profession differ greatly. A person might enter the field to uncover her or his own problems. Another person might have a need to be viewed as an expert. Someone else might have a need to nurture and care for others. Still another might simply enjoy helping others to get more out of life. It is through self-examination and professional training that a helper learns to use beliefs and motivations in the most constructive manner.

SELF-EXPLORATION

To increase your self-understanding and better understand how you react to other people, it might be helpful to consider the following questions:

- What qualities of my personality do I like and dislike?
- What qualities would I most like to change?
- How do I go about solving my problems? Do I seek help from others or try to solve problems myself?
- How do I respond to the problems of friends and relatives? Do I run away? Feel scared?
- Do I feel obligated to find solutions for other people?
- Am I able to control my emotions if necessary?
- How do I show my feelings of love and concern for others?
- Am I able to express positive feelings when this is appropriate?
- What are my most important long-range goals?
- How do I come across to other people?
- Do I feel comfortable in social situations?
- Am I a good listener?
- Can I communicate my ideas effectively?
- What are my motivations for wanting to help others?
- What do I hope to get out of helping others?
- What kind of work activities give me the most satisfaction?

After this initial consideration of your suitability to the helping professions, the next step is to focus on this question: What qualities and characteristics of personality have been shown to be most beneficial in establishing constructive helping relationships?

QUALITIES OF AN EFFECTIVE HELPER

Learning to become an effective helper is not simply a matter of using a correct or proven method. It is very difficult to distinguish between good and poor helper on the basis of the methods used. Rather, quality is measured best by the helper's ability to understand and use his or her own qualities and abilities in the most effective manner.

An effective helper is a product of education, training, and experience. Knowledge alone is no guarantee of success. However, some evidence indicates that certain personal qualities and characteristics appear to be particularly beneficial in the helping relationship. Let's take a closer look at some of these qualities next.

Listening

This is a quality that most people possess in one degree or another. It sometimes implies, however, that a person actually just waits for someone else to finish talking. That person more often than not "listens" by preparing what to say next rather than attending to the speaker.

In the human services field, listening has a special quality. Listening requires a genuine interest in the other person. The helper has to keep wondering, What is this person trying to communicate to me? What is he trying to say about his behavior and his feelings? Often, the helper must listen to both the verbal and the nonverbal messages. The nonverbal messages include the client's facial expressions, tone of voice, posture, gestures, pauses, and silences. For example, if a friend tells you that she feels fine today but her voice is quivering, her speech is unusually rapid, and she cannot sit still or look you in the eyes, you may feel the person is really communicating a very different message.

The art of listening is enhanced by a genuine desire to communicate with others. You may ask yourself whether you are a person who can listen to a friend and really understand what he is telling you. If you are a person whom others seek out to talk to, you most likely possess this quality. Practicing listening will therefore increase your effectiveness in understanding others as well as yourself.

Communicating Effectively

All relationships between people depend on some kind of communication. Through communication people understand and influence each other and learn more about themselves and others. A major task of a human services worker is to establish and maintain relationships with people based on effective communication with others. Effective communication involves expressing yourself through nonverbal and verbal channels. Words and symbols do not mean the same things to all people, and mishaps in communication can cause significant damage to clients. Communication that is comprehensive and clear is basic to effective problem solving. Without good communication, problems cannot be expressed or fully understood, and appropriate solutions cannot be found.

Good communication involves listening effectively and speaking clearly. Can you make yourself understood clearly with others? This may sound simple enough, but often many of us cannot really get our "message" across to another person.

Communication must be sound and easily understandable. This does not necessarily mean using words with fewer than two syllables. It means the helper must respond in terms of the client's feelings and behavior. A person's feelings are always valid and real. Another way to increase your ability to communicate effectively is to focus on "you/me" talk. Effective communication involves you—your feelings, and behavior; and me—my feelings and behavior, rather than a third party (who is not present to represent him- or herself). By using concrete language involving feelings and focusing on you/me talk, you can maximize your abilities as a helper and develop more rewarding relationships as a person.

Empathy

This is one of the most helpful qualities a human services worker can possess. It involves the ability to see things from the other person's point of view, even if you have not shared the same experiences. It means that you can feel and be sensitive about what his or her experiences were like and sense their significance. Sensing another's feelings—that is, expressing empathy—is a natural step toward understanding that person more fully. In a sense, it is like feeling sorry *with* someone because you can understand their feelings and problems, rather than feeling sorry *for* someone. As a helper, you must gain an understanding of how the client views the world. Through this process of sharing the client's world, you are better able to understand his or her experiences and therefore, in a better position to provide meaningful help.

Openness

People tend to open up when they feel the other person is open as well. Of course, a professional helper is there to help the client, not to lay another burden on the client. Openness involves some measure of self-discipline. This implies that the helper is willing to share his or her experiences when this will benefit the client. In the process of helping, you must remember that you are a human being first. If you are open and feel comfortable with yourself, this feeling is usually conveyed to others.

Support

In times of indecision, conflict, and crises, everyone feels a need for support from other people. Even when we are free of problems, we seek out support and encouragement from others. It is a show of neither weakness nor strength to seek out such support but rather a natural condition of human beings.

Are you a person whom friends seek out when they feel such a need? Do you have the ability to give of yourself in this manner? Supportiveness is a very highly regarded quality of a professional helper. Of course, you do not want to offer false hopes or unrealistic expectations to a client but rather communicate faith in the person's own abilities to solve his or her own problems and respect for the client as a human being. Supportiveness also involves conveying a certain amount of reassurance to the person. In another sense, you must be there "in spirit" with this person.

Acceptance

This is a somewhat rare quality but a highly beneficial one for the helping professions. Instead of showing acceptance, some people seem to have a need to pass judgment on others. We do it all the time when we accept or reject people because we judge them to be good or bad. We are almost passing sentence on that person.

As a helping professional, you may be working with people who have done something that you do not like. Say you were counseling an ex-convict who committed rape. Could you effectively help that person if you personally feel that this crime was unforgivable?

Being accepting requires the ability to avoid imposing values and criteria on the other person. This does not mean that you must agree with the client's values. In other words, you can accept the human being as worthwhile without accepting his or her behavior.

WHAT DOES ONE LOOK FOR IN A CAREER?

People are motivated to enter a particular career for a variety of reasons. As previously discussed, there is no single or correct reason. Often, many considerations shape and influence our decision making. Some of these factors relevant to the selection of a career within the human services field are examined in this section.

Income

How much money and resources one desires is a very subjective and personal choice. One person may feel that an adequate income is the ability to afford a primary residence and a second vacation home and have the money to take vacations whenever and wherever he chooses. Another person may feel satisfied with her income if she simply has enough money each month to pay rent and essential bills. Clearly, each individual must assess his or her lifestyle needs and desires and look realistically at the selection of a career in terms of total life satisfaction. Various careers within the human services field offer different levels of income. Of course, many people would like unlimited income, but, as we know, money alone does not necessarily gives us satisfaction in life, and income alone should not be the sole factor in selecting a career.

Status

Status refers to the way we see ourselves and the way in which others and society view us. Society creates and gives more status and prestige to certain professions, jobs, or positions than others. This relates to what a society values as important. Although the idea of status is an artificially created concept, if we perceive it as being valid, then we make it our reality.

A profession that gives off more status does not necessarily mean it also offers more money. For example, a sanitation worker may have a higher salary than a teacher in certain areas, but frequently some people regard teachers as having a higher status. Often a desire for a higher status motivates people to achieve higher goals within a specific career, such as becoming the head of a department or director of an agency.

Status is another means that we have created to evaluate and compare ourselves to others. Some people choose a career to attain a higher status, which then can ultimately become another element of how they view themselves.

Work Satisfaction

Individuals spend a great amount of time throughout their lives being employed. Many get up each morning and actually look forward to going to work because they derive satisfaction from the work they do. Others dread their work and only look forward to their days off. A considerable amount of research has shown us how important it is for our physical and mental health to have a positive attitude, reduce stress, and find satisfaction and purpose to our lives. People who enjoy what they do often are healthier, happier, and more fulfilled individuals. For some, satisfaction with work is actually more important than a higher income doing something they do not truly enjoy. Some are fortunate enough to combine both. Satisfaction and enjoyment in one's work is a critical consideration in choosing a career.

Working Conditions

The work environment is often as important as the environment we create for ourselves in our personal or home life. Research in the field of psychology has shown us how one's environment affects one's behavior and emotions. Many of us spend a great deal of time and effort choosing the right apartment or house and then a lot of time and money making it into something that feels comfortable. We do this because it gives us a sense of satisfaction and pleasure and reflects what we value.

A similar type of consideration should be given to one's work environment. Of course, not everyone can significantly change or modify the workplace to suit individual needs. However, it is worthwhile to give thought to what needs you may have that will impact where you work. To begin to sort out what may be important to you, think about the following questions:

- How much flexibility will I have to change/modify my personal work space?
- Will I have my own office?
- Will I have windows to the outside?
- How do I feel about the physical setting?
- Will I be supervised?'
- With whom will I work?

WHAT DO HUMAN SERVICES ORGANIZATIONS LOOK FOR IN THE SELECTING OF STAFF?

Human services organizations differ from the corporate world in many respects. Selection of staff within the human services field is not solely based on the job candidate's ability to make money for the company, as in most business settings. Human services organizations consider the following aspects of the individual.

Self-Awareness

As previously discussed, your self-knowledge is a valuable personal trait and professional tool within this field. To avoid making value judgments on clients and imposing your worldview onto the client, you must first know yourself very well. Often, questions asked in interviews are designed to evidence the degree of the job applicant's self-awareness.

Values

Organizations, like people, possess a value system. Each human services setting has its particular policies, codes of conduct, and organizational philosophy. For example, some organizations become very involved in clients' personal lives, whereas others define their services differently. Staff are selected based on their personal values and how they might coincide with the values of the organization. Whenever possible, try to gain a sense of the organization and its philosophy prior to an official interview.

Motivation

Many people entering the human services field are motivated by their desire to help others, which is, of course, a solid foundation on which to build.

Because the field involves a diversity of client populations (for example, children, teenagers, adults, elderly) and client problems (such as substance abuse, AIDS, and homelessness), you need to be clear about your motivation for wanting to work with a particular population or agency. Very often the primary question asked of a job applicant is "Why do you want to work here?" It is important for you to be able to consider this issue prior to an interview and be prepared to define your own motives and interests.

Skills/Training

As in any profession, the necessary skill to perform the specific work role is usually a prerequisite for employment. Within the human services field, a variety of specific skills-training programs are available. When working with various client populations or problem areas, the organization will require specific skills. Such may be the case working within substance abuse programs, crisis intervention programs, prevocational training programs, and others. If you are motivated to work in a particular area, it is always advantageous to seek out and acquire specific training.

Education

Some level of formal education is necessary in most areas of the human services field. The type of degree and length of education required vary among the discipline areas. These requirements are provided in detail in the chapters describing each career.

Experience

Very often the difference between getting a job and not getting it is experience. Most human services agencies prefer a candidate to have relevant experience with a similar client population or program. Those individuals desiring to work in a specific area of the field should seek opportunities whenever possible to increase their experience in their area of interest. Those who have little or no paid experience beyond their formal educational training may find that an educational internship or field experience within an educational program can be viewed by some agencies as suitable experience for a particular job. Volunteerism is another avenue to gain experience and provide a prospective employer with some further indication of motivation and ability.

SUMMARY

By now you might have recognized that these qualities overlap. One quality tends to serve as a basis for others. Without empathy, truly understanding someone would be hampered. Without effective communication and listening, showing support would be difficult.

Underlying all these qualities, a sincere desire to help others and a genuine respect for people is a must for the professional helper. The qualities described here in some measure represent the ideal. If you lack some of these qualities, it does not necessarily mean that you cannot eventually become an effective helper. Striving to fulfill your capabilities in these areas is a lifelong goal.

Having thought about the qualities that contribute to becoming an effective helper and exploring your own beliefs, motivations, and expectations, you are now in a better position to consider your more specific career choices.

REFERENCES

Corliss, A. C., & Corliss, R. A. (1998). *Human service agencies: An orientation to fieldwork*. Pacific Grove, CA: Brooks/Cole.

Lock, R. D. (1996). *Taking charge of your career direction: Career planning guide* (Book 1). Pacific Grove, CA: Brooks/Cole.

McClam, T., & Woodside, M. (1994). *Problem solving in the helping professions*. Pacific Grove, CA: Brooks/Cole.

McMahon, S. (1996). *The portable problem solver: Having healthy relationships*. New York: Dell.

Peterson, G. W., Sampson, J. P., & Reardon, R. C. (1991). *Career developments and services: A cognitive approach*. Belmont, CA: Wadsworth.

Schmolling, P., Youkeles, M. & Burger, W. R. (1997). *Human services in contemporary America* (4th ed.). Pacific Grove, CA: Brooks/Cole.

ADDITIONAL READING

Corey, M. S., & Corey, G. (1998). *Becoming a helper* (3rd ed.). Pacific Grove, CA: Brooks/Cole.

DuBois, B., & Miley, K. K. (1999). *Social work: An empowering profession* (3rd ed.). Boston: Allyn & Bacon.

Harris, H. S., & Maloney, D. C. (Eds.). (1996). *Human services: Contemporary issues and trends*. Boston: Allyn & Bacon.

CHAPTER 3

CAREERS AS A GENERALIST WORKER

WHAT IS GENERALIST HUMAN SERVICES WORK?

A generalist in the human services field is one who has not had formal education or earned an academic credential beyond the baccalaureate degree (B.A., B.S., or B.S.W.). Traditionally, a person was considered a professional upon earning a master's degree or doctorate in one of the human service disciplines. There is a growing movement, however, to consider the worker with a two-year and/or a baccalaureate degree as a professional. That aside, the term *generalist* has gradually replaced the title *paraprofessional*, but you will occasionally find *paraprofessional* still used today. Job titles for generalist workers that name the specialty (for example, *social work* or *psychiatric*) and then a level (such as *gerontology aide* or *mental health assistant*) provide other clues as to the worker's role, the types of clients served, and the agency setting.

Generalist or *human services worker* is really a generic term rather than a job title. The National Organization for Human Service Education and its sister organization, the Council for Standards in Human Service Education, draw on the Labor Department's *Occupational Outlook Handbook* for a list of job titles. These organizations are referenced in the "Professional Organizations" section of this chapter, and you are urged to familiarize yourself with their print and electronic outreach. Following is a sampling—not a complete list—of some job titles in which human services workers are employed as generalists:

Adult day care worker	Group activities aide
Assistant case manager	Intake interviewer
Child abuse worker	Life skills instructor
Client advocate	Mental health technician
Community organizer	Outreach worker
Eligibility counselor	Residential counselor
Family support worker	Social service liaison
Gerontology aide	

Why Choose Generalist Human Services Work?

There are good reasons for entering the human services field as a generalist. First, it provides an opportunity for testing a career field before investing a great deal of time and money to prepare for it. In addition, one can gain on-the-job experience before entering advanced training. Second, it provides an opportunity for beginning a career one enjoys while earning a salary. Third, the need for personnel is great and jobs are available in many areas throughout the country. Human services work is among the top ten of rapid-growth occupations, according to the Bureau of Labor Statistics. More than 168,000 human services workers were employed in 1994. Job market information is also provided later in this chapter, along with some electronic and print resources.

Entering the human service field as a generalist does pose some disadvantages. Salaries are low compared with other helpers' compensation. The work is not always exciting or rewarding, and the worker is at the "bottom of the ladder" with regard to choice of assignments or work. There are additional limitations, but if one is determined to work in the field of human services and cannot enter it on an advanced level immediately, these limitations are not overwhelming.

Development of Generalist Human Services Work: Career Trends

Before the 1960s, terms such as *paraprofessional* or *generalist human services worker* were practically unknown. There were hospital attendants who had little, if any, training except in the performance of basic custodial duties. In the late 1950s, mental health professionals recognized that there was a shortfall of professionally trained workers. With the increase in many kinds of human service programs in mental health, education, and community development during the early and mid-1960s, the shortage became grave. Serious consideration was given to earlier recommendations to provide the necessary personnel by developing training programs for new levels of workers. Several programs were developed in the early 1960s that used college students and "indigenous" workers to help provide needed services. Indigenous workers are those who live in the community in which they work and who may also resemble clients in terms of social class, race, or ethnicity. Some workers were also consumers of services and had dealt with the same problems facing the people they were serving. The theory was that an ex-addict, for example, could be very helpful to another addict or a person at risk of substance abuse. The agencies established during the War on Poverty of the 1960s became the largest employers of *paraprofessionals* or *new professionals,* as they were also called. The hiring of indigenous workers also reduced local unemployment and provided workers with career ladders and opportunities to advance by learning new and marketable skills.

Purdue University developed a degree program in 1966 to train mental health or human services workers. Since that modest beginning, more than four hundred colleges have established similar programs. Community colleges offer a two-year associate degree program, and the four-year colleges offer baccalaureate programs. This was, and still is, considered a beginning step toward attaining professional status. The significant increase of mental health personnel trained in these various programs and the recognition of their vital contributions to the provision of services have led to the establishment of organizations (listed later in this chapter) that focus on improving the status, recognition, training, and competence of human services workers.

What Does the Generalist Human Services Worker Do?

It is easier to answer this question by identifying what a generalist does *not* do in the human services field. According to studies, only the prescription and provision of medication are not mentioned as a responsibility. In one form or another and at different levels, the tasks of generalists overlap those of some professional workers. One difference is that tasks are assigned or delegated *by* professionals *to* generalists. For example, a generalist might conduct intake interviews, determine fees, gather information, and serve as a member of a therapeutic team. The professional worker does these things and also provides supervision of subordinates as well as intensive psychotherapy, differential diagnosis, or treatment planning. Overlap in the tasks of two different work roles can lead to tensions between generalists and professionals, particularly in the field of mental health.

Job descriptions don't always mention the kind of custodial and housekeeping work human service generalists may be required to do. We know very few generalist human services workers who do not do some unglamorous work, such as keeping files. Responsibilities of generalists vary according to agency setting, supervisor, and client group. It is also important to know that job titles also vary tremendously. Two mental health therapy aides in different units of the same institution could have different responsibilities. One aide might be assigned primarily to providing custodial care to patients—that is, to make sure they are clean, dressed appropriately, and present at activities. The other aide might lead ward meetings, conduct activity therapy sessions, or contact parents and families. Because these titles and different responsibilities can become very confusing, it is important that you are clear about what duties you will accept and under what job title.

Here are some examples of assignments by title. A drug abuse counselor who has a high school diploma and one year experience in the mental health field interviews drug abusers upon their first visit to a clinic. The primary task of the counselor is to obtain information from and about the client that is required for admission to the treatment program. The information includes address, age, marital status, employment, education, type of drug abuse, length of addiction, size of the habit, family relationships, or reasons for seeking help. The counselor not only is interested in the specific answers but observes and assesses the behavior of the client answering the questions. Does the client look at the counselor? Does the client hesitate before responding? Sit quietly? Give contradictory information? How does the client dress? What is his or her attention span? What level of language is used? This information is given to the treatment team. Getting the client to trust the counselor enough to provide the needed information requires skill, sensitivity, and patience.

Another example of a generalist at work is the social work associate who might work in a home for the aged. The associate meets with newly admitted residents, who often become withdrawn and bitter because they feel rejected, lonely, and worthless. In addition to participating in team meetings and working in treatment and activity therapy programs, the social work associate observes and interacts with residents and submits reports to the treatment team. The focus of the therapy programs might be to help the residents deal with problems of family relationships, self-image, new friends, individual resources, or advantages and disadvantages of living in a home for aged. The associate might in limited instances assume the role of the group therapist when professional therapists are not available to provide these services.

A Day in the Life of a Generalist Human Services Worker

Amy E. earned her B.A. degree in applied psychology/mental health at an Eastern university. She is presently employed in a halfway house serving ten deinstitutionalized mental patients. There are five female and five male residents served by seven staff consisting of a director, assistant director, and five generalists, including Amy, with the title "milieu therapists," who work directly with residents in their real-life situations.

A typical day for Amy might look like this:

9:00–9:30 A.M.: Amy reads the reports of what occurred with the residents during the previous evening and overnight. She notes that John had an intense argument with Dan during the evening and that the anger did not lessen before bedtime. She would keep an eye on both residents and try to help them deal with their anger without hurting each other.

9:30–10:00 A.M.: Amy meets with other staff members to discuss plans for the day. They discuss who will be liaison to job sites and sheltered workshops, who will supervise the making of meals, who will accompany residents to hospital or doctor, and similar assignments.

10:00–11:00 A.M.: Amy meets with John and Dan, whose display of anger is of concern to other residents and the staff. She attempts to help them discuss their feelings toward each other and hopefully resolve their differences before they become a risk to themselves and others.

11:00 A.M.–12 noon: Amy attends a case management meeting with the assistant director. They discuss plans for Judy, a resident who is presently able to enter a sheltered workshop on a limited basis and who must also see her therapist regularly.

1:00–2:30 P.M.: Amy calls and/or visits the different job sites and sheltered workshops in which residents are placed. She meets with supervisors to discuss the problems or progress of the residents. On this day there were no particular problems or signs of noticeable progress on the part of any of the workers.

2:30–4:30 P.M.: Amy meets with the residents assigned to the sheltered workshop to discuss the happenings of the day and any problems they may have encountered. Mary told Amy that she was upset about how the workshop supervisor spoke to her. The group then discussed how Mary might respond to the supervisor.

4:30–5:00 P.M.: Amy writes up her notes on her work with the residents and her perceptions of the resident's progress or problems. These notes will be shared with the entire staff for use in making future plans to help the residents.

Amy clearly is very interested in and enjoys her work. It is a learning experience and could be even more so if there were more (professional) supervision.

How Does One Become a Generalist Human Services Worker?

One may become a generalist worker in the human services simply by obtaining a job in a human services agency without having obtained a graduate degree. To attain higher positions and thus higher salaries and more "psychic income," a generalist must make a substantial investment of time, energy, and money. The higher the position that is sought, the greater the effort required for future training.

The best way to obtain higher positions and salaries is by increasing your competence or effectiveness. This is usually accomplished by successfully completing a training program. There are two major types of training programs. The first is the program established by the institution providing services, such as a mental hospital, nursing home, or social agency. These training programs are provided to help staff members become more effective in their work. This is sometimes called "on-the-job training." Some institutions or agencies also provide training courses for nonstaff members or special groups of individuals who wish to enhance their skills. The programs developed by the service institution focus on the needs of that institution. The courses deal with issues and problems the staff might be facing in their work. For example, if in a children's developmental center the children resist taking part in activities, a course on how to motivate children might be given. The variation of courses and training is great because the needs of the institutions, the staff, and the clients vary so much from institution to institution. The more courses successfully completed, the more competent the worker is presumed to have become and the greater the chance for advancement. Some institutions require every staff member to take part in some training. Other institutions offer courses, and each staff member decides whether to attend. The training programs are usually run by experienced staff members and professional workers.

The second type of training is offered in colleges and universities throughout the United States. According to the *Occupational Outlook Handbook* published by the federal government, during the mid-1990s, 375 certificate and associate degree programs in human services or mental health were offered at community and junior colleges, vocational-technical institutes, and other postsecondary institutions. In addition, 390 programs offered a bachelor's degree in human services.

A brief look at two degree programs might be helpful to the prospective student and worker. Because of the great variety of degree programs in these fields, it would be somewhat misleading to claim that the two programs described here are typical. We suspect, however, that there are many more similarities among the various programs than there are differences, in both philosophy and coursework.

One program offers a two-year associate of science degree in community mental health, and students are strongly encouraged to further their education at least to the baccalaureate level, if not further. The program consists of 21 credits of mental health courses, 18 credits of behavioral science courses, and the 21 remaining credits in liberal arts coursework. More specifically, the seven three-credit courses in mental health include Introduction to Human Services, Aging and Mental Health, Interviewing and Group Leadership Skills, Activities Therapy, Theories and Principles of Psychotherapy, and two semesters of supervised fieldwork in a mental health facility working directly with patients. The mental health faculty provides on-site supervision for the fieldwork courses ensuring the integration of theory and practice. Behavioral science courses include Introduction to Psychology, Developmental Psychology, and Behavior Pathology, in addition to courses such as Introduction to Sociology and Sociology of the Family.

The second program, a four-year human services program, prepares students for entry-level employment in human service agencies. The degree requirements include 48 credits of professional courses, 21 credits of related courses, and the 51 remaining credits in liberal arts courses, including electives. Examples of the professional courses are Counseling, Drug Abuse, Social Service Systems, Aging and Human Services, Mental Health and the Law, and fieldwork in a social service agency. Related courses include psychology and sociology.

These descriptions are brief and at best give only a glimpse of what human services programs can be like. We must emphasize that it is essential to investigate and examine in detail any program you might wish to enter. Try to determine the kind of courses you can choose from to meet your needs. Find out from graduates what they think of the program. Are graduates accepted to advanced programs or sought after by employers? You are the buyer. Examine the service you are planning to purchase very carefully. It is your career and should be handled with care.

LICENSING AND CERTIFICATION

There is at present no licensing or certification program for generalists, although some states do have licensing or registration requirements for specific job titles. Check with the faculty of the program for which you intend to register regarding these requirements. Strenuous efforts are being made to establish certification and program-approved standards for mental health personnel and training programs.

SALARIES

Some salary data can be obtained from the National Organization for Human Service Education, which provides support and identity and networking opportunities for workers and teachers in the human services field. With an acronym pronounced "nosey," NOHSE is listed later under "Professional Organizations." A 1997 NOHSE on-line colloquium described a range of $15,000 to $24,000 for recent graduates of two-year college degree programs in human services, depending on the region of the country and on certifications and licensure in a specialty such as crisis intervention or alcoholism counseling.

Occupational Outlook Handbook salary estimates were $15,000 to $24,000 per year in 1997 for human services workers. For psychiatric aides, the range was approximately $12,000 to $20,000. The handbook, also listed under "References," projects increases in all human service occupations with the single exception of psychiatric aides in hospitals. About one-half of psychiatric aides now work in hospitals, but these positions are declining as hospitals try to contain costs by limiting inpatient psychiatric treatment. However, the decline in inpatient treatment may be slowing; if it does, the job market for this position may slowly change again.

JOB DESCRIPTIONS

Listed here are samples of job opportunities for human services generalists with high school diplomas or two- or four-year degrees. Included in the descriptions are job titles, qualifications, duties or responsibilities, and salaries.

Title: Psychiatric aide I
Location: State mental health facility
Salary range: $6.10 per hour (approximately $12,700 per year)
Qualifications: Training in patient care or six months' experience.
Duties: Interact with patients, assist in cleaning facilities, maintain a
    safe environment for patients, observe and record patient behavior,
    accompany patients to activities, work with groups in socialization
    programs, accompany patients to other areas of hospital or other
    facilities.

Title: Case aide
Location: In-community facility (ICF)
Salary: $7.33 per hour starting salary (approximately $15,000 per year)
Qualifications: High school diploma or GED and at least one year's
    experience working with individuals with developmental disabilities.
Duties: Provide supervision and programming for residents of ICF
    in such areas as self-care, health, nutrition, recreation, socialization,
    community awareness, independent living, communication, self-
    preservation, and behavior management; 40 hours/week.

Title: Social services aide
Location: State Department of Mental Health
Salary range: $20,000 to $22,000 per annum
Qualifications: Associate degree in human services and one year of experience working with adolescents. Additional two years relevant work experience can be substituted for degree. Must have therapeutic crisis intervention training and valid driver's license.
Duties: Crisis intervention/prevention.

Title: Counselor
Location: State Department of Corrections and Mental Hygiene in a large northeastern city
Salary range: $19,000 to $24,000 per year
Qualifications: Graduation from an accredited four-year college with a concentration in psychology, mental health, or social work; two years' experience; passing a written exam.
Duties: Crisis intervention, short-term counseling, court orientation for agency clients; referrals, advocacy; liaison with assistant district attorney and other court agencies; establish contracts and referrals with service providers; maintain records; bilingual English/Spanish desirable; salary dependent on experience.

PROFESSIONAL ORGANIZATIONS

Council for Standards in Human Services Education (CSHSE)
Northern Essex Community College
Haverhill, MA 01830

National Association of Social Workers (NASW)
750 First St. NW, Suite 700
Washington, D.C. 20002-4241
(202) 408-8600
www.naswdc.org

National Organization for Human Services Education (NOHSE)
Tacoma Community College
6501 S. 19th St.
Tacoma, WA 98466-6100
www.nohse.com

REFERENCES

Garfield, S. L., & Bergin, A. E. (1994). *Handbook of psychotherapy and behavior change* (4th ed.). New York: Wiley.

Gartner, A. (1971). *Paraprofessionals and their performance: A survey of education, health, and social service programs.* New York: Praeger.

Russo, R. J. (1983). *Serving and surviving as a human service worker.* Prospect Heights, IL: Waveland.

Schmolling, P., Youkeles, M., & W. Burger (1997). *Human services in contemporary America* (4th ed). Pacific Grove, CA: Brooks/Cole.

Sobey, F. (1970). *The nonprofessional revolution in mental health.* New York: Columbia University Press.

Thomas, K. R. (1993) Professional credentialing: A doomsday machine without a failsafe. *Rehabilitation Counseling Bulletin, 37,* 187–193.

U.S. Department of Labor, Bureau of Labor Statistics. (1998–1999). *Occupational Outlook Handbook.* www.stats/bls.gov/oco/ocos060.htm

CAREERS IN SOCIAL WORK

WHAT IS SOCIAL WORK?

Social work can be defined in many different ways. We define it as a profession that helps people regain and/or improve their ability to live happily, successfully, and fully. In addition, the social worker helps individuals, families, and community groups shape their society so that they can achieve their goals. The social worker does this with the knowledge, skills, and values acquired during professional training.

WHY CHOOSE SOCIAL WORK?

People do not become rich practicing social work. Almost any social worker will tell you that she or he isn't in it for the money. There are other reasons to become a social worker. First, it should be acknowledged at the outset that salaries *are* going up, not rapidly, but steadily enough to stay ahead of inflation. According to the *Occupational Outlook Handbook*, median earnings for social workers with a bachelor's degree (B.S.W.) were $25,000 in 1997; for those with a master's degree (M.S.W.), $35,000. Second, the job market is favorable. *The Occupational Outlook Handbook* projects a faster than average increase in employment of social workers through the year 2006. Other labor market experts are also optimistic regarding job growth in social work, especially with regard to social workers who serve particular client groups such as children and older people. Job prospects are very good as well in particular settings such as hospitals, the workplace (employee assistance programs), and publicly funded halfway houses. And although positions are not always open in all geographic areas, they are usually available for those willing to relocate. A third reason to consider social work is that you will be part of a profession that is recognized as making an important contribution to people and society. If you have a strong desire to help people, social work is a profession that will serve you in your wish to serve others. Fourth, social work provides the worker with a broad range of career opportunities. The prospective social worker can serve almost any population he or she chooses, if not in one community, then in another, and in a variety of settings. You can find social workers in public agencies and private businesses; in hospitals, nursing homes, and clinics; in schools; in police departments and courts; and in private practice. Fifth, this kind of variety provides countless opportunities for the worker to learn about others as well as him- or herself.

DEVELOPMENT OF SOCIAL WORK—CAREER TRENDS

A brief history of how the field developed reveals how the role of social worker has become increasingly professionalized. Today, it would be more appropriate to speak of social worker roles, for with professionalization has come specialization. The history of how the field has developed foreshadows a discussion that continues today among social work practitioners and theorists about professional identity.

In the second half of the 1800s and the early 1900s, a variety of events and social forces created stresses and problems in living, especially for low-income people arriving in the nation's expanding cities from other nations or from America's small towns and rural areas. Stresses were caused by combined effects of population growth, increased immigration, rapid industrialization, World War I, and the Great Depression, among other factors. Problems that resulted included poverty, inadequate housing, child labor, and crime. Many organizations were created to deal with these problems. For example, the Massachusetts State Board of Charities and various departments of public welfare were established to relieve problems associated with poverty. Volunteers, sometimes called "friendly visitors," were the first workers to provide services to the needy. By the early 1900s, some of these volunteers had become paid workers.

Education and training as well as salaries for social workers heralded the professionalization of the field. In that same period, the first social work schools were established. The first mental hygiene clinic for children was started and the first White House Conference on Children held during the early 1900s. Social workers began to work in settlement houses, juvenile courts, and schools. Additional schools of social work were established to meet the growing need for more highly trained workers.

Social workers joined in an ongoing debate from 1880 to 1920 about the causes of poverty, to what degree the poor might be responsible for their own misfortunes, and the obligations of the wealthy and of society in general.

"Scientific charity" was one response to human suffering. This movement was self-consciously modern and examined efforts to relieve poverty in terms of outcomes rather than good intentions alone. Whether they were paid employees or volunteers, however, most social workers came to understand—and assert—that being poor and dependent was not a sign of stupidity or laziness. Social workers shared a growing belief that the intolerable conditions under which people lived and worked were created by social and economic systems rather than by the poor and needy themselves.

After World War I, the professional ideology and focus of social work shifted. A "second revolution" in mental health was triggered by acceptance of the concepts of Sigmund Freud and the medical model of treatment and service in social work. Social workers began to focus on personal psychology rather than the economic and social problems of society as a whole. The causes of problems were sought within the individual. The goal was to get the individual to adjust to external conditions rather than challenge and change these conditions. This became the established approach of social work through the first half of the 1950s.

In the late 1950s, undergraduate programs in social work were established to meet increased demand. Social workers are still searching and experimenting in the hope of becoming more and more effective. Training and practice are based on the perception that every individual is part of many worlds—including family, friends, work, community, and culture—and that professional social workers must be attentive to all of these in their work with clients.

Social workers now work in many capacities—therapist, advocate, case manager, and broker, to name a few—with many different types of clients. Clients vary enormously in terms of their social class, age, and presenting problems or issues, as do the settings in which social work services are provided. During the early history of the field, social work was associated with charity work; today social work professionals work with clients at all income levels. Depending on their income, clients may pay their own fees or be subsidized or have services paid by health insurance. Clearly, it is no longer only the "less fortunate" (that is, the poor) who are served. Yet the public's image of the social worker has been shaped by the origins of social work as charity and philanthropy provided principally by (female) volunteers.

WHAT DOES A SOCIAL WORKER DO?

Perhaps the best way to describe what social workers do is to divide their responsibilities into six major categories: (1) direct practice, (2) supervision, (3) administration, (4) consultation, (5) research, and (6) education. These categories are in no order or priority, and many social workers work in more than one category. For example, supervisors often do direct practice or administration. An administrator might feel it is very important to "keep in touch" with direct practice.

As explained in Chapter 1, managed care has had an impact on all of the helping occupations, social work included. Therefore, this overview of what a social worker does alludes to managed care as a new context in which many social workers must now function.

Direct Practice

Direct practice is the face-to-face contact with those receiving services. A school social worker advises a child who has problems at school. Persons hospitalized with physical illnesses are helped by medical social workers. Their families may also be assisted. As patients get ready to leave the hospital, social workers also participate in discharge planning or aftercare. As the title implies, the psychiatric social worker serves individuals with mental or emotional disorders. Clinical social workers encounter those who have problems in living and generally work in mental health and outpatient clinics as well as in private practice. Social workers also practice in public welfare agencies, correctional institutions, colleges, nursing homes, and senior centers. Because of the wide variety of people and problems, social workers provide a broad range of services and use different techniques and approaches depending on need.

Group services is another area of social work involving direct or face-to-face contact with clients. The social worker may interact with a group of teenagers in a settlement house who are at risk of drug or alcohol abuse. In a Y, a social worker may be helping parents with issues around disciplining their children or step-/blended families. A group of discharged psychiatric patients in an outpatient unit can, with the help of a social worker, learn to cope with the problems they are facing in their families and communities. Social workers in senior centers help groups of older adults plan and participate in activities for therapeutic reasons as well as for enjoyment and expansion of interests and abilities. Social workers deal with clients in social agencies, psychiatric clinics, mental institutions, settlement houses, community centers, senior centers, and nursing homes.

A social worker may function in the role of community organizer to help people in a community improve the conditions and services in their own neighborhoods. The community worker might be sent by an agency or invited by the community to provide help in stemming neighborhood deterioration: inadequate housing, insufficient police protection, low-quality schools or health and recreation services, filthy streets. The community service worker helps organize people in the community and encourages coalition building among organizations such as community councils and welfare organizations in an effort to solve shared problems.

Supervision

Whether in the health field, community work, family work, or criminal justice, social workers often supervise others. A beginning social worker may supervise volunteers. The more experienced worker may supervise graduate students who are placed in the agency for fieldwork experience. There are social workers whose major responsibility is to supervise other social workers. Supervision has two major purposes or goals. One is for the transmittal of knowledge and skills, the educative purpose. The second purpose, administrative in nature, is to ensure that work is performed accurately and expertly within the rules, regulations, and policy of the agency. Supervisors also provide support and resources to help the less senior, less experienced social worker. Supervision usually occurs on a regularly scheduled basis, most commonly for one hour each week, on a one-to-one basis.

Furthermore, it is not only agency rules that must be attended to. With the advent of managed care, supervisors must be cognizant of the rules and procedures of the managed care organization to safeguard the interests of the agency as provider as well as those of clients/consumers.

Administration

Most social workers have some administrative duties, and many social workers become full-time administrators. Agencies, institutions, and programs traditionally have some form of sponsor. The sponsor might be a board of directors for a private, nonprofit agency or a governmental body set up by law. These sponsors usually select an administrator to run the agency or program according to their policies (guidelines). These guidelines might include the kinds of services to be provided and how much money can be spent. The administrator's job is to do everything possible to provide the best service possible. He or she is responsible for hiring personnel, setting standards for performance, composing job descriptions, and monitoring working conditions. The administrator must see that funds are spent wisely and that expenses do not exceed the budget. He or she must be able to design a clear system of communication so that workers and staff know what they and others are doing and how they can help one another be more effective. The administrator makes the final decisions regarding the implementation of policies determined by the sponsors. Administrators and supervisors must have top-notch writing and evaluation skills because, as providers, they are required not only to provide "best practice" interventions but to document and assess outcomes.

Managed care has increased the administrative load of many social workers. It has expanded the roles of others. For example, if managed care places limits on the types of referrals that can be made (such as those to an "out-of-network" psychiatrist), social workers must scramble to secure the needed service from some other agency, serving as a broker on the client's behalf as well as a case manager. In general, managed care has had greatest impact on social workers involved in treatment.

Consultation

This area focuses on helping professionals become more knowledgeable and more effective in their work. A consultant in social work might be asked to give an opinion or information in a courtroom about a person accused or convicted of a crime. A consultant is used because he or she is more objective, expert, or knowledgeable than those advised. A consultant may help an administrator reorganize an agency or department. The social work consultant can have many different kinds of experiences over a number of years or a special expertise in one particular phase of the profession, such as child care.

Research

Research has always been an important aspect of social work. The constant introduction of new theories requires close examination and testing so that they can be used productively in new approaches to social work. Another very important research responsibility is to determine the needs of people, communities, and society. If one can identify the needs, better plans can be devised to meet those needs. Another focus of research is evaluating what has been done. Is a program or a service accomplishing its goals? If not, why? And how might it be improved?

Education

The social work educator helps in the education and training of other social workers as well as research and consultation. Social work educators need to be in touch with the "real world" so that they are aware of changing conditions, problems, and approaches. In addition, social work educators must be familiar with the literature (published research and theory) of the field and attuned to the social issues and policy questions that constitute the context of professional practice.

The next section describes what one social worker actually does. No one job is entirely representative. What is typical of social work in this description is that there is a combination of several different categories of responsibilities.

A Day in the Life of a Social Worker

Gary is a licensed certified social worker with a M.S.W. degree. He works in a large settlement house located in a low-income neighborhood of a midwestern city. Gary was recently promoted to the position of supervisor of the teen division serving boys and girls between the ages of 13 and 17. He supervises two licensed and certified social workers, a dozen club and activity leaders (human service generalists with associate's or bachelor's degrees), and three graduate students in social work. Gary and his staff work in the afternoons and evenings.

A typical day for Gary might look like this:

1:00–2:00 P.M.: Gary meets with his supervisor, the program director of the agency, to discuss plans for the teen division, problems and progress of staff, the status of the groups, and budget issues. Gary also expresses concern about one of his professional staff who is having marital problems; the problems are affecting the quality of his work.

2:00–3:00 P.M.: Gary chairs the teen division staff meeting. The staff and Gary present problems they are having in their work with the teenagers. They explore ways of dealing with the problems and how they might improve the entire program. They discuss the importance of sharing information on individuals and groups that are displaying behavior problems so that all the staff can pool their knowledge and come up with more effective helping strategies.

3:00–4:00 P.M.: Gary has a supervisory meeting with one of the graduate social work students to discuss the student's efforts in helping members of his group limit aggressive behavior at the agency and on the street.

4:15–5:45 P.M.: Gary meets with a co-ed group of older teenagers who are concerned about intimacy and sexuality.

7:00–8:00 P.M.: After dinner, Gary meets with a group of parents who are concerned about drug sales in the neighborhood and the possibility that their own teenage children might get involved in the sale and/or use of illegal drugs.

8:00–9:30 P.M.: Gary meets with the Teen Council, which is made up of representatives of the teen clubs. He listens to their plans, problems, and feelings. He tries to help the council resolve its own problems as well as develop and carry out its plans.

9:30–10:00 P.M.: Gary reviews and organizes the notes he took on the day's meetings and makes an outline of the multipage report that he must complete by the end of the following week. Gary is kept very busy as supervisor of a large program. He enjoys working with teenagers even though at times they are prone to impulsive behavior and resist authority.

How Does One Become a Social Worker?

The title "social worker" is sometimes used loosely to refer to a variety of different jobs held by people with a variety of educational credentials and training. Strictly speaking, the criteria for professional social worker are determined by the National Association of Social Work (NASW). The minimal requirement for being accepted as a professional by the NASW is graduation from a baccalaureate program in social work accredited by the Council on Social Work Education.

Bachelor's of Social Work Program

You should make sure that the social work program to which you are applying is accredited by the Council on Social Work Education. It should not be too difficult to find such a program, as over 400 undergraduate social work programs have been accredited at U.S. colleges and universities. The Council on Social Work Education offers an updated listing of these programs as well as the addresses, phone numbers, and names of individuals with whom you might correspond.

Programs for a bachelor's in social work prepare students for beginning generalist practice. The coursework includes a sound liberal arts background in addition to courses emphasizing the social and organizational contexts of professional social work practice, the values and ethics guiding that practice, and the responsibility and opportunities of continued professional development. Most programs also stress preparation for practice with diverse populations. This is not simply a matter of political correctness. Diversity is taken very seriously by the profession. Programs prepare their students to work with people who are different from them in terms of race, ethnicity, social class, and culture. All accredited programs must include at least 400 clock hours of supervised fieldwork, in which students work directly with clients under the guidance of a professional social worker. Because of the variety of programs in social work at the undergraduate level, we urge the prospective student to explore several programs before selecting one.

The degree and membership in the National Association of Social Workers establishes one as a professional social worker. With regard to one's professional career there are advantages and disadvantages in obtaining the B.S.W. degree. The advantage is that you reach professional status and enter the field sooner than if you waited to earn a master's degree in social work. You can begin earning a living and gaining experience sooner. Among the disadvantages is that the baccalaureate does not command the starting or top salaries that the M.S.W. does. The kinds of positions open to those with the M.S.W. are not always available to those with the B.S.W. In addition, some licensing or registration is limited to M.S.W. degree holders. When the opportunity arises, students should continue their education to obtain the M.S.W. degree. We recognize the need to earn a living often prohibits this step immediately, but it should be seriously considered.

Master's Degree in Social Work

Formerly, the only way to become a social worker was through a master's program. Today, entering an M.S.W. program *without* going through a bachelor's program is advantageous to three groups of students. By not entering a B.S.W. program, the student who is unsure of his or her career goals but wants to "work with people" will have more time to decide whether to become a social worker. Obtaining a liberal arts degree or a bachelor's degree in psychology or sociology can help make that decision. Second, this option may make sense for those students who live in a community where an M.S.W. program is available. The third group of students who can benefit from entering the field via the master's route are those who have long been out of school and have already obtained a bachelor's degree in a non-social work program. Many schools look for such people because the accumulation of life experiences and increased maturity usually produce a highly motivated and often very successful student.

Submitting an application for admission often involves writing an autobiographical statement about significant aspects of your life that led you to a career in social work. Schools look for students who write clearly and creatively. Graduate schools usually require at least a B average in undergraduate work. Schools look for students who have done well in communication skills and English courses as well as political science, history, psychology, and sociology. Excellent letters of recommendation (three are usually required) as well as successful work experience in the field as a volunteer or entry-level paid worker are also important for admission. Some schools still require a personal interview as part of the admission procedure.

There are over 125 accredited M.S.W. programs in the United States. You may want to contact more than one school and obtain descriptions of programs, admission requirements, and costs. Applicants often have a choice of schools, so the more information you have, the easier it will be to make a sound choice. Visiting the school and discussing the program with a faculty member or a school representative can also be of great benefit.

The coursework offered by graduate schools of social work varies substantially, even though any and all of the programs you should consider will have been accredited by the Council on Social Work Education. An annual *Directory of Accredited BSW and MSW Programs* is available for a nominal fee from the Council on Social Work Education. Many schools emphasize the common elements of direct practice; some focus on the knowledge aspects of the profession. The introduction of information and knowledge from other disciplines has increased. For example, a course on Issues in Social Work might include material on social work and family policy (including new federal welfare reform), the most recent updates of the NASW code of ethics, and social work and the law. Course material on the history of social welfare and an emphasis on social policy is usual. Some schools have introduced systems theory in their curriculum. All programs are required to increase course content addressing diversity. This variety of programs, which is a healthy sign for social work education and for the profession, makes it essential for you to determine which program meets your needs and will hold your interest.

Doctoral Programs in Social Work

Programs offering the D.S.W. or Ph.D. degrees offer advanced-level training to social workers who want to pursue leadership positions in social policy, administration, or college teaching. A doctor of social work program usually takes at least four years to complete and requires a book-length dissertation research study as well as coursework.

Cyber Sources of Information

Many colleges and universities have their own Web sites and post information about their undergraduate and graduate social work programs, including curriculum and sample program plans. Professional organizations, including, of course, the NASW, have their own home pages. Many provide career information and job postings on-line. The home page of the Council on Social Work Education provides a full statement of its criteria for program accreditation and lists accredited programs alphabetically by school and state. There are chat rooms and on-line magazines such as *The New Social Worker Online* (www socialworker.com) for new and prospective social workers; others can be accessed via keywords and search engines. So start surfing!

Licensing and Certification/Credentials

A growing number of states license, certify, or register social workers. The basis for these procedures varies from state to state. Most states require an exam for certification or licensing and registration. All of them use one or more levels of the American Association of State Social Work Boards (AASSWB) exams. Educational requirements also vary from state to state. In some instances, two years of college might be sufficient; a master's degree is required in others. Certification, licensing, and registration in all states is a goal of professional organizations such as the NASW. It is seen as a form of protection for the profession and the consumer and is used in many instances as a basis for determining salary.

Credentials—as awarded by the NASW—require a degree, supervised experience, professional references, adherence to a professional code of ethics, and passing an examination. The purpose is to certify competence and professionalism beyond a college degree or state license. NASW credentials include the ACSW, which certifies membership in the Academy of Certified Social Workers for independent, self-regulated practice; School Social Work Specialist (SSWS) for providers of social services and mental health services in school settings; Qualified Clinical Social Worker (QCSW), for which requirements include 3,000 hours of postgraduate supervised clinical experience; and the NASW's highest professional clinical certification, the diplomate credential (DCSW).

SALARIES

Salaries in social work range from $25,000 for the social worker with a B.S.W. to well over $38,000 for an experienced social worker with an M.S.W. Length and type of experience and job descriptions are basic to the determination of salaries. Typical job descriptions with requirements and salaries follow. Some advertisements highlight fringe benefits and the advantages of working and living in a particular area. Salaries vary, depending on the location of the job. Salaries in large urban areas are often higher than those in rural areas or smaller cities. Federal employment pays more than state or local government jobs or, in many cases, private agencies.

JOB DESCRIPTIONS

Title: Psychiatric social worker
Location: Community mental health center, outpatient unit
Starting salary: $30,000 to $35,000 depending on ACSW certification and experience. Above-average fringe benefits program.
Qualifications: M.S.W. Broad-based psychotherapy skills with all age groups required, including group therapy skills. Consultation and emergency skills helpful.

Duties: Individual and group counseling, working with transdisciplinary team. Flexible hours, day and evening shifts. Some crisis intervention work.

Title: Social worker
Location: Family service agency
Salary: Position currently funded at $28,000 per year and benefits
Qualifications: M.S.W. degree and a mature individual.
Duties: Handle a diverse caseload including counseling with the elderly, children, families, and adults. Flexibility and dedication to work with a small innovative agency required. The position also offers an opportunity to work with family life education and eventual supervision of graduate students. The area offers an ideal climate with close access to the Gulf of Mexico.

Title: Social worker IIIs and IVs
Location: County Department of Social Services, Children's Services Division
Salary: SW III: $2,163 to $2,630 per month; SW IV, $2,321 to $2,822 per month
Qualifications: BSW for SW III; M.S.W. or M.A. in psychology, sociology, or related field required for SW IV.
Duties: Maintain cases and perform investigations

PROFESSIONAL ORGANIZATIONS

Council on Social Work Education
1600 Duke St., Suite 300
Alexandria, VA 22314-3421
(703) 683-8080
www.cswe.org

National Association of Social Workers
750 First St. NE, Suite 700
Washington, D.C. 20002-4241
(202) 408-8600
www.naswdc.org

American Association of State Social Work Boards
400 South Ridge Parkway, Suite B
Culpepper, VA 22701
(800) 225-6880; (540) 829-6880
www.aasswb.org

REFERENCES

Addams, J. (1910). *Twenty years at Hull House.* New York: Macmillan.

American Association of State Social Work Boards. (1997, updated annually). *Social work laws and board regulations: A state comparison study.* Culpepper, VA: Author.

Council on Social Work Education. (1997, updated annually). *Directory of colleges and universities with accredited social work degree programs.* Alexandria, VA: Author.

Leiby, J. (1979). *A history of social welfare and social work in the United States.* New York: Columbia University Press.

Lubove, R. (1965). *The professional altruist: The emergence of social work as a career 1880–1930.* Boston: Harvard University Press.

Richmond, M. (1895). *Friendly visiting among the poor.* New York: Macmillan.

Schmolling, P., Youkeles, M., & W. Burger (1997). *Human services in contemporary America* (4th ed). Pacific Grove, CA: Brooks/Cole.

Trattner, W. (1974). *From poor law to welfare state: A history of social work in America.* New York: Free Press.

U.S. Department of Labor, Bureau of Labor Statistics. (1998–1999). *Occupational outlook handbook.* www.stats/bls.gov/oco/ocos060.htm

CAREERS IN COUNSELING

WHAT IS COUNSELING?

According to the American Counseling Association (ACA), counseling is a career that is designed to prevent, diagnose, and treat mental, emotional, physical, or behavioral disorders. Counselors can also help people overcome a specific crisis and/or problem and help clients develop goals and objectives that contribute to a healthy lifestyle. Over the last 20 years, counseling has become an extremely diverse field of study. Counselors are trained to offer support and advice to individuals and groups who are seeking help in areas such as alcohol and drug addiction, child abuse, establishing career and academic objectives, and seeking advice regarding marital, family, and spiritual issues.

Unlike psychologists, counselors place little, if any, emphasis on long-term analysis and psychodynamics. Counselors prefer to offer alternatives and possible solutions to specific problems of daily living. An addiction counselor, for example, may suggest a 12-step program to an alcoholic and offer support and advice during the recovery period, or a marriage counselor may choose to see a couple and suggest ideas and skills that will enable the couple to achieve a happy and satisfying relationship. The ultimate goal of counseling is to encourage cognitive and behavioral change. More specifically, it is the responsibility of the counselor to help his or her client identify maladaptive behavior, learn healthy decision-making skills, and develop skills that prevent problems from reoccurring.

WHY CHOOSE COUNSELING?

This career offers the deep satisfaction that comes from helping others achieve a secure and satisfying lifestyle. In addition to personal satisfaction, counselors have a variety of academic degrees and employment opportunities to choose from. Counselors, based on their individual strengths and level of interest, can pursue an A.A., B.A., M.A., or Ph.D. in a number of different specialties. In addition to academic degree programs, many colleges and universities also offer certificate programs in specialized areas of counseling such as drug and alcohol abuse and marital and family counseling.

For students who prefer to pursue a degree, the field of counseling offers specialized areas of study. Several of these specialties include, but are certainly not limited to, community counseling, career counseling, gerontological counseling, marriage and family counseling/therapy, rehabilitation counseling, school counseling, mental health counseling, and pastoral counseling. Students interested in these areas of specialization can contact the ACA at (703) 823-9800 or visit its Web site at www.counseling.org/ for further information.

Professional counselors help people grow cognitively, emotionally, socially, and educationally in a variety of work settings. Here are some typical work settings:

- Community centers
- Mental health agencies
- Hospitals
- Rehabilitation facilities
- Nursing homes
- Schools
- Colleges/universities
- Private businesses
- Private practices

Counseling is a broad and expanding field. The beginning counselor can look forward to opportunities that are both challenging and financially and emotionally rewarding.

DEVELOPMENT OF COUNSELING—CAREER TRENDS

Man's inhumanity to man is nowhere more evident than in the treatment of physically and emotionally disabled persons. In terms of the physically disabled, the killing or banishment of people with physical disabilities and deformities was quite common in earlier civilizations. In medieval times, it was believed that the will of God was expressed in the crippling of certain persons. The disabled were simply abandoned to beggary or ridicule. Even in our more enlightened age, people with disabilities are victims of outright discrimination in regard to jobs and educational opportunities.

For the most part, large-scale rehabilitation and counseling are historical latecomers. Serious attempts to help the blind, disabled, and mentally challenged were not made until the 1800s. In these early efforts, there was a tendency to simply accept the dependent status of people with disabilities. They were provided with the essentials for survival, but no real attempt was made to rehabilitate them.

The rehabilitation movement in this country gained ground after World War I by showing that many disabled servicemen could be restored to active, useful living. During the 1920s, attention shifted to the plight of workers who were disabled by industrial accidents. A federal/state rehabilitation program for disabled workers was launched. Meanwhile, private organizations assumed responsibility for helping persons with specific disabilities such as blindness or retardation.

The need for qualified counselors became pressing after Congress passed a rehabilitation program for World War II veterans. Highly trained counseling psychologists were too few in number to fill the need. It was at this time that the job title "rehabilitation counselor" began to make its appearance. In 1950, there were only about 1,500 rehabilitation counselors, most employed in state vocational rehabilitation programs. By 1976, the number had soared to nearly 19,000, reflecting increased federal/state funding rehabilitation.

Presently, the need for rehabilitation and counseling services is enormous and continues to grow at a rapid rate. In 1990, the federal government estimated that there are close to 50 million people with some form of physical, cognitive, or psychological disability. With this in mind, the federal government passed the Americans with Disabilities Act. This law was specifically designed to create and finance programs that will provide rehabilitation services to members of our disabled population.

Another major advance in social attitudes toward disability took place during the turbulent 1960s. For the first time, socially disabled persons including criminals, the poor, children with learning, behavior, and emotional problems, and addicts became eligible for rehabilitation services. The idea was no longer to restore persons to a former level of functioning but to help those who had not developed adequate skills in the first place. In 1963 the federal government passed the Community Mental Health Act, which in effect changed the role of rehabilitation and school counseling in the United States. By passing this law, the government mandated specific services for a number of target populations. Groups such as students, the elderly, and victims of substance abuse would now be entitled to a wide range of diagnostic, treatment, liaison, and follow-up services. In addition, counselors were now encouraged to expand their treatment and rehabilitation roles to intervention and prevention. It is no longer sufficient or acceptable to merely treat the child with a disability, the inmate in prison, or the executive with a cocaine addiction. Today, counselors are encouraged to get involved in programs and services that will prevent and minimize the impact of certain emotional and physical disabilities.

Just as the demand for teachers has picked up markedly from the doldrums of the 1970s and 1980s, the market for persons trained as general counselors also shows definite improvement. According to national, regional, and state surveys, career opportunities are expected to improve through the year 2006.

Today the job market for community, career, mental health and gerontological counselors appears to be good. Counselors who specialize in these particular areas with an emphasis on prevention and early intervention can look forward to a variety of employment opportunities.

For rehabilitation counselors, the future outlook appears particularly good. Presently between 65 and 75 percent of second-year master's students find either full- or part-time positions in paid fieldwork or internship settings. Many professionals in the field believe that the need for qualified rehabilitation counselors will continue to grow. Advances in medical technology, the increase of individuals who will require rehabilitation counseling, and new legislation requiring equal employment rights for individuals with disabilities will only enhance the need for rehabilitation counselors in the future.

Because rehabilitation has grown from a career that deals with vocational counseling to a career that involves personal, social, and interpersonal aspects of a person's life, trained rehabilitation counselors have the option of seeking employment as school, college, and agency general counselors. The high level of training required for rehabilitation counseling compares favorably with that received by persons trained for school or career counseling alone.

The outlook for school counselors also appears to be good. Because of school counselors' expanding concerns (for example, drug and alcohol abuse, crisis intervention, child abuse, teen pregnancy, suicide), the need for experienced and qualified counselors is going to grow. Limited funding and budgetary restraints, however, will to some extent limit the hiring of much needed counselors.

What Does the Counselor Do?

The role that the counselor takes when working with a client depends on the type of problem that is being addressed as well as the work setting. One of the most attractive features that counseling has to offer is its diversity. In addition to different areas of specialization and work settings, counseling also offers the beginning counselor the opportunity to work independently and/or on an interdisciplinary team with other human service professionals. Depending on their area of specialization, counselors can work with children, teenagers, young adults, adults, and seniors in an individual and/or group setting. One of the goals of counseling is to help others reach their individual goals. In their attempt to help others achieve this goal, counselors have several different roles to choose from. They can (1) counsel and work with individuals who have a problem and are seeking *treatment,* (2) design and conduct workshops for "at-risk" individuals in an attempt to *prevent* a problem from occurring, or (3) work with certain target populations who are experiencing the early onset of a particular problem and develop a *crisis intervention* program. The role that counselors play in their clients' lives can also be nontherapeutic. Many counselors want to help others but choose to do it in the nontraditional role of client advocate. Many people who are in need of help are not aware of the type and scope of services that are available to them. Client advocates in a way become the voice of the client. They educate the client, help them apply for services, and often fight for their clients' rights.

As we move closer to an interdisciplinary approach to mental health, it is essential that counselors understand that they will be an important member of a team. As a team member, they have a responsibility to help their client reach their full potential in life. In addition to choosing what roles they will play in a client's life, counselors also have the opportunity to choose the type of work setting they would like.

As you can see, the many choices available to the beginning counselor can seem overwhelming. An outline of specialties and suggested work settings are listed, followed by a brief discussion of several popular areas of interest.

COMMUNITY COUNSELING

Counselors who specialize in community counseling focus on a variety of social and community-oriented problems. Community counselors work with individuals and groups who are seeking help in (but certainly not limited to) areas such as domestic violence, drug and alcohol abuse, teen pregnancy, homelessness, and child abuse.

Their role and responsibilities can also vary depending on the type of problem and client they are working with. Substance abuse, for example, can be a fairly typical problem for community counselors. In fact, substance abuse has become so common that many community counselors decide to make it an area of concentration while they complete their graduate studies and eventually specialize in substance counseling when they earn more advanced degrees. Most counselors agree that counseling substance abusers is often a difficult and frustrating experience. Usually during the first few counseling sessions, the counselor learns that substance abusers are insincere, full of broken promises, and often contemptuous of authority figures. The experienced counselor knows that before any meaningful progress can be made the counselor must establish trust and mutual respect between client and professional. Once this is accomplished, the counselor and client will discuss the client's need to develop an alternative lifestyle that includes regular employment, a new circle of friends, and new relationships. As the sessions continue the counselor and client will also discuss and explore issues such as interpersonal relationships, family dynamics, nutrition, and peer pressure. The goal of counseling in this type of situation is to offer support, guidance, and help the client develop skills that will facilitate healthy lifestyle decisions. Counselors help their clients realize that new friends, a different environment, and steady work and income bring both self-respect and the respect of others.

Counselors who have an interest in this area of specialization can look forward to working in mental health agencies, hospitals, community outreach centers, and the human resources department in many large companies.

Other areas of concentration that students may want to investigate as extensions of community counseling or as areas of specialization in and of themselves are career counseling, gerontological counseling, and marriage and family counseling/therapy. Let's take a closer look at these sample areas next.

Career Counseling

Traditionally, career counseling entailed working with a client who was looking for employment. Today, however, career counseling has evolved into a comprehensive and specialized area of counseling. Typically, the career development counselor will evaluate a client's strengths and weaknesses, assess and evaluate skills and special abilities, and explore what the client would like to get out of a particular career and what they feel they have to offer.

Economics and emotional needs are explored as well as the importance of socialization and desired geographic area. In addition to traditional counseling techniques such as establishing rapport with the client, the career counselor must be skilled in the administration and evaluation of vocational tests.

Career development counselors work in community/mental health agencies, high schools, colleges, and many large corporations. They work not only with individuals who are seeking a new career but also with those who have secure jobs. Career counselors believe that people need to be informed of the continual and rapid changes of the modern economy. Career counselors who work for large corporations may, for example, organize workshops and seminars designed to help employees understand what these changes are and how to prepare and adjust to them.

Gerontological Counseling

The problems that our elderly population face can often seem overwhelming, typically including the loss of spouse, friends, and other family members. These feelings of loss might also pertain to their job and home environment. In addition to loss, the aging process also means change. Seniors' bodies change (impaired vision, hearing, and mobility), as do their relationships and socialization with family and friends over time. Children grow to depend less on their parents and friends, and family sometimes move away, causing a void in the elderly person's life. The impact of these losses and changes will almost always have a negative effect on an elderly person's self-image and self-worth. Contrary to how many people view the elderly in U.S. society, many are not inferior or incompetent; in fact, many have the ability to adjust to change and continue leading active and meaningful lives.

The counselor's role in an elderly person's life can be extremely useful. The counselor must first assess the client's strengths and weaknesses. The counselor must also help the client identify, cope, and adjust to a wide variety of feelings. For example, an elderly woman who has just lost her husband or child may feel depressed and guilty. The counselor can help the client learn that she is not responsible for life and death situations and explain that she has a responsibility to herself to accept her sadness and begin to form new relationships and perhaps develop new roles in life.

Recent research has discovered that support and guidance are useful tools in helping elderly individuals overcome guilt, fear, anxiety, and depression, and in some cases tolerate the effects of dementia. Useful counseling techniques that have proven to be effective with the elderly include (1) reality orientation, especially for those individuals who are experiencing some disorientation with person, place, and time; (2) remotivational training, for individuals who need to develop new interests and activities; and (3) reminiscing, with the goal of helping the elderly remember the important aspects of their lives in the hope that they will feel some importance and meaningfulness when they evaluate their lives.

Counselors work in nursing homes, senior citizen centers, hospitals, and community clinics. In addition to working with individual clients, the experienced counselor also designs and organizes support groups and works closely with family members. Family members need to learn that it is important to reinforce independence and activity. All too often family members will encourage inactivity and consequently a life of loneliness and isolation.

Counselors can help their clients go back to school, get new jobs, or find comfortable homes. For those that cannot lead independent lifestyles, counselors can take an advocacy role. Counselors can take an active role in terms of helping the elderly person find certain needed services (for example, meals-on-wheels, visiting nurse, social security benefits).

Marriage and Family Counseling/Therapy

Unlike other forms of counseling, the marriage and family counselor does not work with one individual. During marriage counseling, the counselor will work with a husband and wife (and, if necessary, with one member of the couple for a certain period of time); during family counseling, the counselor will meet and work with immediate family members and, if necessary and relevant, members of the extended family.

The marriage and family counseling session always begins with an intake interview. Here, the counselor obtains as much information as possible. Each member of the group is asked to submit information about different aspects of their lives. Information pertaining to income, career, education, psycho-social history, and health will be used to understand each individual member of the group. This background information may also help the counselor understand why certain problems exist.

With this information, the counselor will now give all members of the group an opportunity to express what they think their problem is. Sometimes members of the group will agree as to what the problem is, and other times, they may express different points of view. One client might say that the issue that has them upset is a financial matter, whereas another may say that they are unhappy with their sex life. At this point, the counselor will give each member a chance to express their feelings and then they will begin to develop a group understanding of how they will approach the problem and/or problems.

Despite the expressed problem, the experienced counselor knows that before any compromise or change can occur, the counselor must help clients achieve a meaningful level of mutual trust and respect. When appropriate, the counselor will help the couple or family to learn useful communication skills and an insight into each other's feelings and needs. If successful, the counselor can now deal with specific issues and offer possible suggestions and recommendations.

Marriage and family counselors usually work in mental health clinics or private practice. They use several different techniques in the course of their work. Role playing, for example, is a typical technique. In role playing, members of the group change roles; a husband will take the role of his wife, and the wife takes the role of her husband. The goal of this exercise is to help the individual clients gain an insight and understanding of how it feels to be the other in creating situations. Audio- and videotapes are another useful technique. By taping sessions, clients have an opportunity to see and hear how they sound and look when they interact with others. Frequently, this objective perspective helps clients see themselves from a different point of view. Counselors find that this is a useful technique to use when a client is resisting looking at him- or herself realistically. The counselor hopes, for example, that when an angry client sees and hears his level of aggression and how people react during an angry episode, he may be more willing to learn how to change and deal with anger in a more constructive manner.

REHABILITATION COUNSELING

One of the main goals in rehabilitation counseling is to help the client make a realistic estimate of limits imposed by the disability. In many cases, the counselor is faced with the client's refusal to recognize the seriousness of the problem. For example, a construction worker may deny that his cardiac condition requires a change to a sedentary kind of work. Other clients may completely give up on life. An individual who is an outpatient may feel too anxious to consider any type of employment. In each case, the counselor helps the client make a realistic appraisal of what he or she can and cannot do. A good relationship between the two helps attain this goal.

During initial contacts, the counselor generally reviews the client's school experience, job history, hobbies, and interests. The counselor listens attentively and tries to conduct the session so that the client will gain insight. If indicated, the counselor might arrange for psychological testing to supplement the information already available. Testing provides information about the patient's intelligence, level of academic achievement, and personality traits. Aptitude tests give an idea of how well the client would do at clerical, mechanical, numerical, or other tasks. The client is observed during the testing. It is obviously important if the client shows extreme anxiety, irritation, or discouragement while working on a difficult task.

Some rehabilitation centers are equipped with shops where patients can try various activities such as carpentry, electronic assembly, drafting, clerical work, and sewing. By being able to actually accomplish a new task, the client gains the confidence that accompanies success. These work sample programs also help the client build up tolerance for prolonged activity. Some disabled persons know how to do a job but can only work for an hour or two. The counselor encourages the client to build up enough tolerance to meet the requirements for at least part-time employment.

The counselor explains the rehabilitation program to the client's family, suggesting various ways they can help. The family members are sometimes just as unrealistic as the client in coming to grips with the disability. For example, in the case of disabled children, the parents usually have to be persuaded to let the children do more on their own. Sometimes, the parents of a child with a mental disability have to overcome their shame about the child's limited capacity. If the family members are not happy with the rehabilitation plans, they may sabotage the entire process.

When the client is ready, the counselor begins the final phase of the rehabilitation process: placement in the community. To be successful at placement, the counselor keeps up good relationships with employers and community agencies. The experienced counselor knows the local job market and can find positions for people with serious disabilities. Clients who are unable to compete in the job market may be placed in a sheltered workshop. Here limited-ability workers can earn money for doing productive work, usually on a piecework basis. For example, a sheltered workshop may do the job of assembling ballpoint pens for a local manufacturer. Although paid less than the minimum wage, these workers derive satisfaction from their earnings. Even a modest paycheck can mean a lot to someone who has never worked before.

If at all possible, the counselor should schedule follow-up interviews to discuss any problems that might have come up in the placement. Perhaps the client is not getting along with fellow workers or having a problem with transportation to and from the job. Whether the problems are deeply psychological or practical in nature, the counselor tries to find a solution. The relationship between client and counselor may continue for months or years.

SCHOOL COUNSELING

School counseling is a unique specialization. It takes the principles of school counseling and offers the beginning counselor the opportunity to choose from one of three subspecialties: elementary, middle/junior high, and senior high school. Counselors who work with children and adolescents focus their attention on the personal, social, and academic aspects of their clients' lives. The school counselor must have an understanding of the stages of human development as well as environmental problems, community issues, and family dynamics. In addition to helping their clients with behavioral/academic issues, school counselors also provide services that include drug and alcohol prevention groups, conflict resolution, and crises intervention (for example, after a suicide attempt).

Counselors who specialize in school counseling can work with individuals and/or small groups and particular types of populations. Within school settings, for example, counselors may choose to work with teenage substance abusers, children who have been physically abused, or victims of domestic violence.

The goal for these and similar groups is to offer support and guidance. Counselors help the client identify their needs, develop the skills necessary for achieving mutually agreed-on goals, and learn various coping mechanisms for a variety of problems. Encouraging clients to share their experiences and express their feelings, the counselor works toward improving the clients' self-image and self-worth. The counselor positively reinforces positive traits and encourages clients to make healthy choices and decisions.

School counseling has become an extremely broad field of study. School counseling is no longer limited to working with teachers and parents. Today's counselor must not only have experience working with a host of diverse problems, he or she must be able to work with a team of specialists. School counselors often consult with psychologists, social workers, physicians, and community leaders in their attempt to facilitate the academic and emotional development of their students.

In today's world, the school counselor must have the knowledge and expertise that it takes to help a 15-year-old female who is failing her courses, having difficulty adjusting to changes at home, and taking drugs as a way of dealing with her feelings. In this and other typical situations, the school counselor must know how to assess and evaluate the problem, have the skills to counsel the child, know how to utilize outside agencies, and make suggestions to other school staff members and parents.

School counselors primarily work in public or private schools with children in grades K–12. School counselors are also found in colleges, prisons, alternative school programs, the military, private industry, and sometimes in community outreach centers.

The population and type of problems the beginning counselor chooses to work with will decide where he or she works. For example, the counselor who wants to work with young children with emotional and learning disabilities will want to consider working in a private or public elementary school. For the counselor who wants to work with teenagers who are victims of substance abuse or domestic violence, he or she will want to look toward working in a high school or community outreach center. Opportunities in the high school environment also include career and vocational counseling. Counselors in this setting also have an opportunity to design and participate in various prevention and intervention programs.

Beginning counseling students who want to work with older students in a college or university atmosphere should pursue graduate training in student affairs practice in higher education. Counselors who pursue this specialization are interested in working with individuals who are in the process of making many lifestyle changes. College counselors help students with emotional issues, separation anxiety, career choices, and interpersonal relationships.

School counselors can also choose jobs that do not require individual or group counseling. Individuals can work in public or private agencies as student advocates. Individuals who choose to be student advocates are interested in helping students attain the services that they deserve. Student advocates are also dedicated to building a social and educational system that is fair and just to all people.

MENTAL HEALTH COUNSELING

Mental health counselors work with clients or patients who suffer from an emotional disability. They are trained to work with individuals of all ages and cultural backgrounds and trained to deal with a wide range of problems. Mental health counselors help individuals who suffer from problems such as schizophrenia, manic depression, suicide, eating disorders, and anxiety panics. Mental health counselors work in mental health agencies, community halfway houses, hospitals (inpatient and outpatient centers), and nursing homes. They work with clients/patients independently and in groups. Often, mental health counselors are also members of an interdisciplinary team (psychologist, psychiatrist, social worker, nurse). As a member of the human service team, the counselor plays an important role in contributing information for the treatment of the client/patient.

The role that the counselor plays in the clients'/patients' lives varies from individual to individual. The counselor may help the client/patient deal with some family issue, find a job, or provide support and sensitivity when the client/patient is feeling depressed or frustrated.

A specialization in mental health counseling is one good example of client advocacy. As mentioned earlier, some counselors choose to take a nontherapeutic role in their attempt to help others. The mental health counselor has that opportunity. They can fight for their clients'/patients' rights. They can help them receive the best treatment possible while they are confined to a facility, apply for economic aid, or find a place to live once they leave the facility.

PASTORAL COUNSELING

Essentially pastoral counseling incorporates the principles of counseling with spirituality. They may address many of the more general topics already described (for example, personal relationships, family and work issues) within the framework of a client's religious values. Pastoral counselors do not need to be a minister, priest, or rabbi. Often pastoral counselors are dedicated professionals who address a client's spiritual beliefs in the counseling session.

Like other counselors, pastoral counselors can work with individuals, couples, and groups. They work in a variety of religious organizations, community centers, and mental health agencies.

A Day in the Life of a Rehabilitation Counselor

After graduating from college with a B.A. in psychology, Luisa worked for two years as an interviewer for the Division of Vocational Rehabilitation in her home state. This experience encouraged her to seek advanced training in rehabilitation counseling, and she eventually earned her master's degree in this field. She now works for a private agency that provides rehabilitation and other services to the visually disabled. Here is a brief account of a typical day in her professional life.

9:00–10:30 A.M.: Luisa attends a seminar at the agency along with other staff members. The main speaker is the agency's medical consultant. Discussion centers around the damaging effect of certain types of diabetes on the retina and other parts of the eye.

10:45–11:30 A.M.: Luisa has a counseling session with a young man she has seen once before for an initial interview. He is a graduate student in musicology who is progressively losing his sight. At this point, the client is not ready to discuss the specifics of a rehabilitation plan. He has not fully accepted the verdict of his doctors that his disorder cannot be reversed. Luisa helps him struggle with the question of why he was singled out for this affliction.

11:45 A.M.–1:15 P.M.: This is the day selected for a once-a-week, informal luncheon conference. Also present are a counseling psychologist, a social worker, another rehabilitation counselor, an occupational therapist, and the director of the agency. There is animated discussion about the possibility of establishing a training program in computer technology for the blind clients.

1:30–2:30 P.M.: Luisa counsels a middle-aged woman who has always had limited sight. The client, a capable homemaker, wishes to enter the job market now that her children are grown. Toward this end, she has been working hard to learn typing and transcribing from tapes. Luisa helps her explore her fears of working outside the home.

2:30–3:30 P.M.: Luisa counsels a young man who has been blind since birth. She and the client discuss the client's desire and anxiety regarding his return to school. The client expresses his desire to attend a four-year college and get his degree. Luisa reassures her client and focuses on reinforcing his strengths and resources, explaining that it is important for the young man to work on self-confidence during their counseling sessions.

3:30–4:00 P.M.: Luisa confers with a social worker about the potential sources of funds to help pay for a client's college tuition.

4:00–5:00 P.M.: Luisa devotes the last part of the day to handling correspondence, writing progress notes on her clients, and filling out agency forms.

Luisa is very satisfied with her job. She appreciates the easy, informal atmosphere that prevails at this small agency. In particular, she enjoys the one-to-one contact with clients, though sometimes she feels frustrated by the time that must be devoted to staff meetings and paperwork.

How Does One Become a Counselor?

Although not mandatory, a two-year graduate program that focuses on an area of specialization such as school counseling, rehabilitation counseling, or marriage and family counseling/therapy is strongly recommended. Recent statistics show that six of ten counselors have a master's degree. A few colleges offer introductory courses in counseling at the undergraduate level, but these courses are not intended to equip a student to become a licensed or certified counselor. With a B.A., a student might be able to get a job as a counselor trainee or employment interviewer, but more employers are requiring graduate training for certain positions.

Students should plan to attend a four-year college with a major in behavioral sciences. You should also include courses such as human development, abnormal psychology, and sociology in your course of study. If you know what area of specialization you wish to pursue or the target population you want to work with, you should take courses that would provide important background information. For example, any course providing some basic medical background will be particularly useful for students specializing in rehabilitation counseling. Courses in child development will be particularly useful for students who want to work with children. Some command of a second language such as Spanish is considered very useful in this field. At least a year before graduation, write to the Office of Human Development Services for a recent list of schools receiving training grants from the federal government. Also, send for catalogs from all of the schools you might possibly be interested in attending. If you need financial help to pursue your training, ask the program director for information about student aid. Most graduate schools can arrange aid for students who meet certain requirements.

Before choosing one of the many programs that are available, students interested in counseling should contact the Counsel of Rehabilitation Education or the National Board of Certified Counselors for a list of approved programs of study.

Graduate Training

Currently, more than 124 accredited institutions offer graduate training in various areas of counseling. The two-year graduate programs include study of behavioral sciences and the cultural and psychological aspects of a variety of disabilities.

There is also an emphasis on clinical skills such as interviewing and group leadership. The theories and techniques of counseling are taught in the classroom and then applied in supervised practice. During this internship, the student works with real clients and learns how to be supportive while at the same time encouraging the client to move toward greater self-reliance and self-fulfillment. The program is rounded out with practical information about community resources and, in the case of rehabilitation counseling, some knowledge of physical and occupational therapy.

The amount of coursework and length of internship vary according to the area of specialization. Community, career, gerontological, and school counseling degrees usually require 48 credits plus an internship, compared with marriage and family counseling/therapy and mental health counseling, which require approximately 60 credits plus an internship.

Again, the beginning student should contact the American Counseling Association for more detailed information regarding degree fulfillment.

Licenses and Certification

Licensing and certification for counseling depend on the individual requirements of the state and city that the counselor plans on working in. Currently, 45 states and the District of Columbia have some type of professional credential for the practice of counseling (Alaska, Hawaii, Minnesota, Nevada, New York, and Pennsylvania have no formal licensing laws at this time). Although each state has its own requirements, the general requirements for state certification include (1) a graduate degree in counseling from an accredited school, (2) successful completion of the National Counselor Exam (administered by the National Board of Certified Counselors), and (3) supervised clinical experience (for example, 300 supervised clinical hours over a two-year period is generally the norm). Once you have completed graduate training, contact the American Counseling Association (www.cecp@counseling.org; see "Professional Organizations") regarding certification information that pertains to your specialization.

Rehabilitation counseling follows a different set of certification requirements. Once a field with little professional status, this specialization has greatly developed and will increasingly specify requirements for employment, training, and certification. The Commission on Rehabilitation Counselor Certification has recommended a set of standards for certification. The certified rehabilitation counselor (CRC) has met minimum standards of training and experience. Those with CRC status take part in a program of continuing education to ensure consistent competence. At present, certification is not generally required for employment. As this field matures, however, one may assume that holding CRC status will help in both advancing and obtaining new positions. The history of new certification levels in any field shows that once established, the best people in the field seek to quality for certification.

SALARIES

As always, salaries depend on training, experience, duties, location, and other factors. As a rule, the federal civil services pay somewhat higher salaries than state or county agencies. Counselors who work for the federal government can begin at a GS-9 level with a starting salary of $30,000 a year and over time can increase to a GS-11 with a salary of $36,000 a year.

The entry salary range for a rehabilitation counselor with a master's degree is $23,000 to $35,000. For substance abuse counselors, the range is $12,000 to $24,000, with the average being approximately $17,000. For school counselors with a master's degree, the beginning salary is between $20,000 and $25,000. In the private sector, career counselors who work for large corporations will earn between $25,000 and $33,000 per year. Career counselors also have the opportunity to become private consultants and earn up to $100 per hour.

JOB DESCRIPTIONS

A good way to learn more about salaries, duties, and qualifications of counseling is to look at job advertisements. For this field, the best sources of such information are personnel departments of each state. Agencies of the federal government, such as the Veterans Administration, are also good sources. Private agencies devoted to helping people with disabilities, such as the American Foundation for the Blind, will also be helpful. Here are some typical job advertisements.

Title: Rehabilitation counselor
Location: A large private agency devoted to helping children with
   disabilities
Salary range: $23,000 to $35,000

Qualifications: A master's degree in rehabilitation counseling, plus one year of vocational counseling.

Duties: Determine clients' eligibility for rehabilitation; obtain medical and social information; organize and design new programs and provide advice to program directors and other counselors.

Title: Substance abuse counselor
Location: Metropolitan drug rehabilitation center
Salary range: $17,000 to $23,000
Qualification: Associate's degree in human services and certification in drug counseling (CDC).
Duties: Conduct intake interviews; individual and group counseling; work closely with neighborhood school staff.

Title: School counselor
Location: High school in a midwestern state
Salary range: $37,000 to $44,000
Qualifications: Master's in school counseling and two years' experience working with adolescents.
Duties: Interview and counsel students with learning and emotional disorders; make recommendations to school staff; organize teen support groups; establish rapport with parents; establish working relationship with community agencies.

Title: Counselor
Location: Urban nursing home
Salary range: $19,000 to $25,000
Qualifications: An undergraduate degree in social/behavioral sciences; experience with the elderly a plus.
Duties: Conduct admission interview with patients and families; conduct individual and group counseling; obtain social and medical background information; assist staff members with difficult counseling problems; provide direct service to some difficult cases.

Title: College counselor
Location: Small undergraduate college in northeastern city
Salary range: $28,000 to $32,000
Qualifications: Undergraduate degree in psychology/sociology; certificate in crisis intervention a plus.
Duties: Work in student counseling office; work with walk-in students who require immediate counseling services; help students find part-/full-time employment; organize support groups for freshman student body.

Title: Vocational counselor
Location: Vocational rehabilitation center in a midwestern city
Salary range: $34,000 to $36,000
Qualifications: Master's degree in rehabilitation counseling plus two years of experience in a rehabilitation setting.
Duties: Work with physically disabled population; evaluate clients' skills; assist clients with job preparations; make appointments and provide transportation to job sites.

Title: Mental health counselor
Location: Midwestern state college
Salary range: $2,191 to $2,829 per month (ten-month position with full benefits)
Qualifications: Master's degree from an accredited counseling program.
Duties: Must have knowledge and experience in the following: psychologically, cross-cultural counseling, group leadership and facilitation, ethical standards and practices.

Professional Organizations

American Association for Marriage and Family Therapy
1100 17th St. NW
Washington, D.C. 20036

American Association for Pastoral Counselors
9504-A Lee Highway
Fairfax, VA 22301

American Counseling Association
5999 Stevenson Ave.
Alexandria, VA 22304
(800) 347-6647
www.counseling.org/

American Mental Health Counselors Association
AMHCA Central
P.O. Drawer 22370
Alexandria, VA 22304

American Rehabilitation Counseling Association
5999 Stevenson Ave.
Alexandria, VA 22304

American School Counselor Association
5999 Stevenson Ave.
Alexandria, VA 22304

Council for Accreditation of Counseling and Related Educational
    Programs
American Counseling Association
5999 Stevenson Ave.
Alexandria, VA 22304
(703) 823-9800, ext. 301
www.counseling.org/cacrep
E-mail: cacrep@aol.com

Federal Research Service, Inc.
243 Church St., Suite 200 W
P.O. Box 1059
Vienna, VA 22183-1059

National Board for Certified Counselors
3 Terrace Way, Suite D
Greensboro, NC 27403
(910) 547-0607
www.nbcc.org
E-mail: nbcc@nbcc.org

Council on Rehabilitation Counselor Certification
1835 Rohlwing Rd., Suite E
Rolling Meadows, IL 60008

REFERENCES

Allan, W. S. (1967). *Rehabilitation: A community challenge.* New York: Wiley.
Benjamin, L., & Walz, G. (1989). *Nine for the 90's: Counseling trends for tomorrow.* Charlottesville, VA: Caps.
Bowe, F. (1980). *Rehabilitating America.* New York: Harper & Row.
Collison, B. B., & Garfield, N. (1996). *Careers in counseling and human services* (2nd ed.). New York: Taylor & Francis.
Courtland, C. Lee. (1995). *Counseling for diversity: A guide for school counselor and related professionals.* Boston: Allyn & Bacon.
Kottler, J. A., & Brown, R. W. (1992). *Introduction to therapeutic counseling* (2nd ed.). Pacific Grove, CA: Brooks/Cole.
McDaniels, C. (1989). *The changing workplace: Career counseling strategies for the 1990's and beyond.* San Francisco: Jossey-Bass Social and Behavioral Science.
Nugent, F. (1990). *An introduction to the profession of counseling.* Columbus, OH: Merrill.

Oberman, C. E. (1965). *A History of vocational rehabilitation in America.* Minneapolis: Denison.

Ogg, E. (1979). *The rehabilitation counselor.* (Public Affairs Pamphlets, 381 Park Avenue South, New York, NY 10016.)

Patterson, C. H. (1980). *Theories of counseling and psychotherapy* (3rd ed.). New York: Harper & Row.

Rehabilitation counselor. (1982). Moravia, NY: Chronicle Guidance Publications.

Toch, M., Perry, P., & Baxter, N. (1997). *Opportunities in counseling and development careers.* Lincolnwood, IL: VGM Career Horizons.

Tyler, L. E. (1969). *The work of the counselor.* New York: Appleton Century Crofts.

Walz, G. R., Gazda, G. M., & Shertzer, B. (1991). *Counseling futures.* Charlottesville, VA: Caps.

SOURCES OF ADDITIONAL INFORMATION

Newsletters

For information on how to obtain these newsletters, contact the American Counseling Association, 5999 Stevenson Ave., Alexandria, VA 22304.

- *Adult Development and Aging News*
- *Child, Youth and Family Services Quarterly*
- *Rehabilitation Psychology News*
- *Psychology of Addictive Behaviors*
- *Psychology in Mental Retardation and Developmental Disabilities*
- *Psychopharmacology Newsletter*

Journals

Additional information regarding counseling journals of the American Counseling Association can be obtained by calling (800) 633-4931 or visiting www.counseling.org/journcat.htm

- *The Career Development Quarterly*
- *Counseling and Values*
- *Counselor Education and Supervision*
- *Elementary School Guidance & Counseling*
- *The Family Journal*
- *The Journal of Addictions & Offender Counseling*
- *Journal of Counseling & Development*
- *Journal of Employment Counseling*
- *The Journal of Humanistic Education and Development*
- *Journal of Mental Health Counseling*

- *Journal of Multicultural Counseling and Development*
- *The Journal for Specialists in Group Work*
- *Measurement and Evaluation in Counseling and Development*
- *Rehabilitation Counseling Bulletin*
- *The School Counselor*

CAREERS IN PSYCHOLOGY

WHAT IS PSYCHOLOGY?

The best way to define psychology is to divide this broad field into two general areas. One is the scientific and systematic study of human and animal behavior and, some might add, mental and emotional processes. About one-third of all psychologists describe themselves as *experimental psychologists*. This means that they do basic research in specialties such as learning, thinking, sensation, and personality. Experimental psychologists are interested in gathering data that helps us understand issues and questions such as how much of our behavior is inherited and how much of it is influenced by the environment, and why people seem to remember certain pieces of information and forget others.

Psychology can also be defined as an applied science. *Applied psychologists* use the knowledge and skills of psychology in a practical way—that is, to solve human problems. Students interested in pursuing a career in psychology have over 20 different specialties to choose from. The majority of students, however, tend to lean toward careers in clinical, counseling, and school psychology. About two-thirds of all psychologists work in applied specialties such as clinical psychology.

Clinical psychologists devote themselves to the study and treatment of disturbed or maladaptive behavior and are trained to conduct research or teach, consult, and supervise. They work with individuals and groups in a wide variety of settings, including medical and psychiatric settings, public school systems, juvenile correction centers, rehabilitation centers, geriatric institutions, and university psychology departments.

In addition to the specialties discussed in this chapter, several others also entail helping other people. Industrial or organizational psychology, for example, involves problem solving in the workplace. Social psychology studies how an individual's attitudes and behaviors are influenced by others in the environment. Students may also consider a career in community psychology. This specialty, which began in the early 1960s, focuses on social and environmental problems such as drug abuse, homelessness, crime, violence, and teen pregnancy. Rather than working in a laboratory or with individuals in a private office, community psychologists are part of an interdisciplinary team who work with and in the community.

WHY CHOOSE CLINICAL PSYCHOLOGY?

Clinical psychology offers the prestige of an established profession, a wide range of interesting duties, and good financial opportunities. Although not in short supply, clinical psychologists (particularly those with doctorates) can look forward to a favorable job market during the next decade. The newly graduated Ph.D. should be able to find a position, although not always in the geographic area of first choice. Established psychologists are usually able to choose how much time to devote to various professional activities such as teaching, clinical practice, and research. In addition, private practice offers additional satisfaction both in terms of helping others and in the financial sense. Today, however, with the growth of managed care systems, the financial opportunities for psychological evaluations and psychotherapy are not as lucrative as they were ten years ago. HMOs have placed strict financial limitations on the number of visits and the amount of money they are willing to reimburse patients for each visit. With this in mind, the beginning professional should anticipate limited additional income from private practice.

DEVELOPMENT OF CLINICAL PSYCHOLOGY—CAREER TRENDS

The roots of clinical psychology go back to the mid-1800s when scientists first attempted to measure various psychological traits, abilities, and skills. The development of the first intelligence test was a major step forward in accurately measuring individual differences in mental capacity. The test measured a person's ability to learn, memorize, and grasp complex ideas, as well as many other mental capacities. It was found that test scores predicted a child's performance in school with impressive accuracy. In fact, the first practical use of these tests was to identify schoolchildren who could not be expected to keep up with a normal class. When the first psychological clinics were established at the turn of the century, psychologists were asked to assess children with school problems. With the development of personality tests, psychologists soon began to branch out into other settings such as mental hospitals and clinics.

During World War I, the military called on psychologists to develop tests to measure the abilities of draftees. The famous Army Alpha Test measured abilities such as arithmetic, vocabulary, and understanding of instructions. Nearly two million men were tested before the end of the war on this and other tests.

After World War I, psychologists continued to work in hospitals and clinics. In many of these settings, the clinical psychologist reported test results to medical superiors. Few clinical psychologists held doctoral degrees in those days. The team approach gradually became the pattern followed in most mental health settings. The psychiatrist was the team leader, whereas the psychologist tested and sometimes provided therapy of an educational or remedial kind. The social worker was responsible for conducting family history interviews and contacting other community agencies. It was not until after World War II that psychiatric domination of the team was seriously challenged by nonmedical professionals.

World War II provided the push for major growth of clinical psychology. With psychiatrists in short supply, psychologists were assigned to military psychiatric units to treat troubled GIs. Thousands of emotionally disturbed veterans were discharged and entitled to the services of the Veterans Administration (VA). The VA launched a program to support training of additional mental health personnel. Paid internships were made available to graduate students in clinical and counseling psychology.

The growth of clinical psychology tended to sharpen conflicts within the field of psychology. By 1949, nearly half of the Ph.D.s in psychology were awarded to clinicians. This alarmed academic psychologists who feared that they would soon lose their traditional control of university psychology departments. The academic psychologists believed that psychologists should be devoted to pure research and scholarship. They opposed premature attempts to put psychological knowledge to practical use. Power struggles between the two factions occurred in many universities. A conference was held in Boulder, Colorado, to clarify the role of clinical psychology. It was agreed by the leadership that the clinical psychologist was to be a psychologist first and a clinician second. In other words, the graduate student was to be trained primarily as a research-oriented scholar with some additional training in a clinical setting. This was the scientist-professional model that prevailed for about two decades.

In recent decades, serious dissatisfactions were expressed from time to time with the so-called Boulder model. Many graduate students complained of an overemphasis on academic and research concerns in their training. They essentially wanted and were asking for more training in the clinical-practical aspects of their work. In response to this demand, a new kind of professionally oriented program was introduced in 1968 called the doctor of psychology

(Psy.D.) program. Unlike traditional Ph.D. programs, this new program does not require a dissertation and substitutes additional practical training. More details about this development are given later.

Clinical psychology is now one of the most popular specialties within psychology, accounting for approximately 35 percent of all doctoral degrees. During the last three decades, clinical psychologists decisively broke out of the psychiatrist-dominated team approach and found new roles in private practice, clinical research, and university teaching.

The role and status of clinical psychology will continue to change. Several psychologists, for example, have already entered training programs that will enable them to prescribe medication to their patients. With the support of the American Psychological Association (APA), states such as Louisiana and Georgia have already presented bills to their state legislatures that will eventually allow psychologists with three years' experience, 300 hours of specialized training, and a year of supervised experience to prescribe medications for treating mental disorders.

In addition to these recent developments, many psychologists are redefining their goals as mental health specialists. While many psychologists continue to *treat* mental disorders, others are either expanding their interests toward intervention or abandoning the traditional treatment approach entirely. According to a recent APA Presidential Miniconvention, psychologists are beginning to "get out of their offices and into the community to alleviate problems that face urban families." Increasingly, psychologists are choosing to work as part of an interdisciplinary team of health care professionals as a way of addressing the needs of society and the community.

Perhaps the most dramatic development that the field of clinical psychology has had to respond to is the recent influence of the managed care movement. Traditionally, clinical psychologists have had the opportunity to make clinical judgments and financial arrangements with their patients and clients. In many ways managed care has forced clinical psychologists to examine new approaches to the traditional treatment plan approach. According to Jean Spruill, Ph.D., who is the director of a psychological training clinic at the University of Alabama, "clinical psychology has become a business and therapy is the product. . . . Psychologists must consider treatment costs and determine the best care for the money." Clinical psychologists are also now being advised to develop a background in administration, management, and marketing skills.

Clearly, clinical psychologists are finding themselves in a rapidly changing world that is slowly advocating change and diversity. If clinical psychologists are to survive in a health care system, they need to deemphasize their role as independent mental health specialists and look toward developing the skills they will need to work effectively as a health care provider.

What Does the Clinical Psychologist Do?

In addition to the traditional task of psychological testing, the clinical psychologist does psychotherapy, counseling, and research. Some clinical psychologists accept faculty positions in a college or university where they conduct basic research as well as teach courses. In addition to salaried employment, many clinical psychologists also maintain a private practice devoted to treatment, testing, and counseling. As the profession has advanced, clinical psychologists have assumed additional administrative responsibilities. It is, for example, not unusual for a clinical psychologist to be an administrator in a large social agency such as a community mental health program. The range of activities of the clinical psychologist has greatly expanded, and we will examine in detail some of these in the next sections.

Psychological Testing

The request for testing may come from any of several sources. For instance, a judge might want to know whether an accused defendant knows right from wrong, or a psychiatrist might request an estimate of a patient's potential for suicide. Testing is often done when some important decision has to be made concerning the person in question.

In clinical practice, particularly in psychiatric settings, a patient is given a battery of tests that includes an intelligence test, projective tests, and some measures of motor coordination. Once the testing is complete, the psychologist scores the tests, interprets the data, and writes a report of the findings. The goal is to come up with an overall description of the personality and to make recommendations concerning future treatment of the patient.

Research

Psychologists receive more training in research methodology then do other mental health professionals. The term *research* refers to the process of seeking information through the use of case studies, theoretical papers, surveys, and experiments. Clinical psychologists predominately conduct research pertaining to abnormal states such as extreme anxiety, depression, psychoses, and addictions. They are also responsible for many studies of assessment and treatment.

Psychotherapy

The desire to do psychotherapy is probably the strongest motive of most beginning clinicians. It is the reward that justifies the long academic grind. Doing psychotherapy involves helping others in a way that brings prestige and income to the helper. Beginning therapists usually bring a great deal of enthusiasm to the work, but as time goes on, therapists realize that there are definite limits to what can be accomplished with psychotherapy. Some clients cannot be helped at all. Others can benefit only a little. The experienced clinician accepts realistic limits to the power of therapy and learns to apply time and effort to cases in which significant benefits can be expected.

Counseling

There is a close, overlapping relationship between counseling and psychotherapy. The distinction is essentially one of emphasis. Counseling usually involves helping the client make important life decisions, whereas psychotherapy focuses on helping the client change undesirable or self-defeating behaviors. Counseling aims to put the client in the right environment. For example, the counselor helps people with career choice and school or marital problems. In each case, the client may be contemplating an important change in one of these areas. In actual practice, it is unrealistic to make a hard and fast distinction between emotional problems and the problem of choosing a path in life. The process of choosing a career is often loaded with emotional overtones. For example, the parents of a young adult might be exerting pressure to make a choice that the young person does not feel is right. Or perhaps the parental choice might be a good one, but the young person rejects it out of rebellion.

Counseling Psychology

We have been talking about counseling as a process somewhat distinct from psychotherapy. Now, let us focus on counseling psychology as a career field in psychology. There are graduate programs in counseling psychology comparable to those in clinical psychology. There is, of course, considerable overlap in these two programs of instruction.

The training of the counseling psychologist emphasizes interviewing skills. The counselor is trained to establish rapport with the client, highlight critical information during the session, and clarify the nature of the problem. In addition, the counseling psychologist is an expert on certain types of psychological tests. For example, aptitude tests are useful in predicting whether a certain client has the ability to do well in a particular job, school, or career. Interest tests provide measures of the kinds of activities that the client enjoys. Personality tests may also provide useful information; if the client is mild mannered and submissive in temperament, he or she may not do well in a selling job. The counselor is also expected to gather information about occupations, careers, and schools. The process of counseling involves putting together the information from all of these sources to help the client make a reasonable choice.

Many counseling psychologists are employed by colleges and universities where counseling centers offer help with personal and career problems. A college student away from home for the first time might come for help with feelings of loneliness and not "fitting in." Another student may be confronted with academic failure and will seek help to try to understand the problem. Some counseling psychologists are employed in hospitals, rehabilitation centers, and community counseling agencies. It is not true that counselors work only with relatively normal clients. However, when they do work with seriously impaired patients, the emphasis is somewhat different than that of the clinical psychologist. The counselor emphasizes helping the person adjust to work and educational settings. In general, counseling psychologists pay special attention to persons in transitions such as adjusting to college, a job, or to divorce and remarriage.

School Psychology

The school psychologist promotes children's social and intellectual development. This may include consulting with teachers regarding classroom behavior problems, administering standardized tests, and developing special programs for the intellectually and emotionally challenged student. For a variety of legal and practical reasons, the school psychologist does not engage in formal psychotherapy with children. One reason is that this would represent an undue investment of time in a single student. The school psychologist is generally busy dividing his or her time between several schools in a geographic area. If therapy is indicated, the psychologist generally refers the child for treatment to a mental health facility in the community.

A student who wishes to become a school psychologist may seek graduate training at one of three levels. The *psychometrician* specializes in the administration and scoring of psychological tests, particularly intelligence tests. Usually, he or she is supervised by a school psychologist and is expected to write a report about the results of testing. Thirty graduate credit hours are generally required to qualify as a psychometrician.

A *psychoeducational specialist* has finished 60 or more graduate credit hours and is trained not only in testing but in various kinds of helping activities such as conferring with teachers and advising students. Some colleges award a professional diploma (P.D.) or a degree as educational specialist (Ed.S.) to those who have completed work beyond a master's degree but do not yet have a doctorate.

The *doctoral level* is the highest level of training for school psychologists. The first graduate from a doctoral program in school psychology was in 1958, a comparatively recent date. The field has grown rapidly in popularity in recent years. The doctoral programs in this area vary in type of degree offered. Some offer a doctorate in education (Ed.D.); others offer a Ph.D. in school psychology. In addition, a few schools are now awarding the Psy.D. degree in school psychology.

Community Psychology

Community psychology is a relatively new field of interest that takes certain psychological principles and applies them to the needs of the community. Contrary to the traditional therapeutic approach of clinical and counseling psychology, community psychology focuses on helping people effectively cope with existing problems in the community and how to avoid and/or minimize these problems from occurring. Community psychologists work in community, government, and mental health agencies. Usually they are members of a inter-disciplinary team of professionals dedicated to helping members of the community help themselves. By combining various research techniques (conducting surveys and observations) with their counseling skills, community psychologists identify a particular problem, design and develop a community-based intervention program that effectively deals with this problem, and supports and teaches members of the community the skills necessary for preventing this problem from reoccurring.

Students who are interested in pursuing a career in community psychology should be dedicated to gaining the knowledge and acquiring the strategies for promoting social change. Graduate and undergraduate programs in community psychology focus on helping the student develop the methodological skills necessary for working with community and human service organizations. These programs also introduce students to the principles of prevention and intervention. As government and community organizations emphasize the need for a new and innovative approach for dealing with drug abuse, domestic violence, and teen pregnancy, community psychology is quickly becoming a respected and popular field of interest.

A DAY IN THE LIFE OF A CLINICAL PSYCHOLOGIST

Sam is a clinical psychologist who was recently awarded a Ph.D. by a large university in the Midwest. He is employed by a state mental hospital located near the capital city of his home state as a staff psychologist in an acute admissions ward. The patients are all males who have recently suffered serious breakdowns involving some loss of contact with reality. Many of the patients on this ward are confused, agitated, and highly emotional.

What follows is a brief description of a typical day in Sam's professional life.

9:00–9:30 A.M.: As usual, Sam begins his day with a visit to the nursing station. He talks to the charge nurse about several incidents that took place during the night. One patient assaulted another during an argument about stolen money. No serious injury was involved. Because Sam is not treating either patient, no intervention on his part is needed.

9:35–10:35 A.M.: Sam attends the staff meeting with a team leader of the ward, who happens to be a senior psychologist. Also present is the psychiatrist who is primarily responsible for medication of patients on this and another ward, a social worker, a psychiatric nurse, and two mental health therapy aids. Discussion focuses on a 38-year-old male schizophrenic who feels strongly that he is ready for discharge. Various members of the team express doubt about the patient's readiness to go back to the community. Sam is asked to administer a battery of psychological tests to help judge the patient's degree of contact with reality.

10:30–11:20 A.M.: Sam conducts psychotherapy with a young, streetwise male patient with a history of multiple substance abuse. During the session, Sam focuses on the patient's hostile attitudes toward various members of his family. Unless these negative feelings lessen, it seems unlikely that the patient will be able to live at home again.

11:30 A.M.–1:00 P.M.: Sam supervises two psychology interns who are learning the rudiments of testing under Sam's direction.

2:00–3:00 P.M.: After lunch, Sam administers an intelligence test to the patient discussed at the earlier meeting. He plans to administer personality tests including the Rorschach ink blot test on the following day.

3:00–4:10 P.M.: As usual, Sam reserves the latter part of the afternoon for his written work. He puts the finishing touches on the report of a patient tested several days ago. Then, he makes some notes on his therapy patients.

4:15–5:00 P.M.: Sam confers informally with the senior psychologist about a research project on which they will collaborate. Essentially, it is a continuation of Sam's thesis research on thinking processes of schizophrenic patients.

It goes without saying that Sam is involved in informal contacts with patients and staff at various times during the day and that he has occasional phone conversations with other professionals. Basically, Sam likes his position at the hospital. However, he believes that there is an overemphasis on medication at the hospital. He would like to see more in the way of group and individual therapy, with increased time spent in therapeutic activities. In general, he feels the patients spend too much time sitting around watching daytime TV programs.

How Does One Become a Clinical Psychologist?

Because psychology is one of the most popular college subjects, it is not difficult to select a college or university that offers an undergraduate major in psychology. However, undergraduate programs vary greatly in quality. The B.A. does not qualify the student to become a licensed clinical psychologist, so it is important to look ahead to graduate school. Be sure that the college you choose has a good track record in regard to its students being admitted to graduate school.

Undergraduate training for a career in psychology usually consists of a basic liberal arts program with a major in psychology. The student generally minors in sociology or the biological sciences. A grasp of algebra is necessary, and courses in statistics, computer science, and research methods are excellent preparation for graduate training. As some graduate schools require competence in a foreign language, it may be helpful to include Spanish, French, or German in the program. Among psychology courses, the student invariably takes developmental, abnormal, and experimental psychology because these classes nurture an aptitude for research.

Graduate Training

Students who are interested in becoming a licensed clinical psychologist *must* earn a doctoral degree from an accredited university and take the licensing exam in the state that they choose to work or practice in. The most desirable kind of training is provided by doctoral programs accredited by the American Psychological Association (APA). Write the APA (see "Professional Organizations") for an up-to-date listing of approved graduate programs in clinical, counseling, and school psychology. The competition is intense. The successful candidate needs an outstanding undergraduate academic record, good recommendations, and satisfactory scores on the Graduate Record Examination and the Miller Analogies Test. Students with less than a B average in college grades and below-average test scores are unlikely to be accepted. It also helps if the student has done some volunteer work in a clinical setting.

The typical Ph.D. program requires four to five years of graduate study. The initial training emphasizes the scientific basis of psychology. Initially, students study basic psychological processes such as perception, learning, and motivation. Later, the student takes more advanced psychological courses. This is followed by the internship, which consists of supervised experience in a clinical setting. The final step is usually the dissertation or thesis, which represents an original research study. For information regarding APA-approved graduate programs, contact the American Psychological Association (www.apa.org/ed/clin.html; see also "Professional Organizations").

Clinical Internship

Academic training, though essential, is not enough to produce a skilled clinician. The clinical internship provides the experience of working with people in a clinic or a hospital. The training is typically one year long, beginning in the third year of graduate study. It may be full-time for one year or spread over several years on a part-time basis. The intern does testing, therapy, and counseling with actual cases under the close supervision of a senior psychologist. The student prepares written reports and is also expected to contribute to case conferences. In other words, the intern does the same kind of work as other staff members but under close supervision.

The internship is usually taken in clinical settings with no formal connection with the graduate school. The training centers are usually well-established psychiatric hospitals and clinics. The American Psychological Association evaluates various facilities and publishes a list of approved internships. Some internships are taken at on-campus psychological clinics under the control of the graduate school. Campus clinics may, however, lack the resources, variety of patients, and range of staff interests that are found in psychiatric settings. Some clinical psychologists believe that the profession will not become fully independent until internships are conducted in clinics controlled by psychologists rather than psychiatrists. Meanwhile, some of the best opportunities for learning are provided by psychiatric agencies.

For more information regarding APA-approved internship placement, contact the APA at www.apa.org.

The Dissertation

The dissertation, an original research project, is a basic requirement for the Ph.D. Although there is variation from school to school, we can outline the general procedure. After deciding on a research topic, the candidate selects a faculty member to chair the dissertation committee. When the committee approves the project, perhaps requiring certain improvements or additions, the student is free to perform the research and collect the information or data. The vast majority of dissertations in psychology now involve some form of statistical or experimental study. The research is typically derived from ongoing research being conducted by faculty members.

Once the data are collected, the student drafts the report on the project, including the theories that were tested, the methods employed, and a discussion of the findings. The final report may be 100 or more pages long. As the student prepares the manuscript, it is submitted chapter by chapter to the sponsor (a faculty member who serves as an adviser about the dissertation topic and process), who returns it with comments, suggestions, and criticisms.

The final meeting of the committee is called the defense of the thesis. The members ask questions of the doctoral candidate about any aspect of the thesis. One may challenge the methods used, whereas another may raise questions about the validity of the conditions. If the committee approves the thesis, the candidate becomes a full-fledged Ph.D. If there are significant criticisms of the work, the candidate might be required to make major revisions. It is extremely rare that outright rejection occurs at this late stage.

The Doctor of Psychology Degree (Psy.D.)

Many graduate students in traditional Ph.D. programs are unhappy about the dissertation requirement and the heavy emphasis on research. The new doctor of psychology degree is designed to appeal to students who are interested in therapy, testing, and the clinical aspects of the work. This new program emphasizes clinical training and does not require a doctoral dissertation. The number of Psy.D. programs has steadily increased, and there is no doubt that this degree is here to stay.

The Ed.D. Degree

The doctor of education (Ed.D.) is another type of doctoral degree earned by psychologists. The Ed.D. is a professional degree awarded by graduate schools of education. The focus is on schools and educational matters. Often little original research is required. This degree is not usually held by clinical psychologists, although a few APA-approved programs in school psychology lead to the Ed.D. degree. Most Ed.D.s are earned by persons who contemplate working in a public school setting or for a college or university. They often work as senior counselors in school or college guidance centers or use this degree for some other phase of the student personnel field.

The ABD Psychologist

The psychologist who has met all the requirements for the Ph.D. except the dissertation is known informally as an ABD ("all but dissertation"). The employment outlook for ABD psychologists depends on the financial status of various institutions and agencies. Agencies faced with economic cutbacks may not always be able to afford the competitive salary range of the Ph.D.

psychologist and turn to an ABD psychologist as a way of saving money and hiring a skilled professional at the same time. Once employed, the ABD psychologist operates under a slightly inferior status. Promotional opportunities and salary increases are limited. Because advancement often depends on the doctorate, the ABD psychologist is under pressure to complete the dissertation.

Too many ABDs in every field take years to complete their dissertation and earn their doctor's degree. Many get so involved in a job that they fail to allocate time to finish their studies. Others are employed in a city far from their home university and find needed contacts difficult to make. Many others get married and find that family commitments and short-term economic needs make it difficult to break away for the life of a scholar.

The Master's-Level Psychologist

There are over 200 terminal master's degree programs in psychology. These programs are "terminal" in the sense that they do not go beyond the master's degree. They usually require one or two years of graduate study, some practical clinical experience, and, sometimes, a master's thesis based on a research project. Students thinking about entering a master's degree program should carefully consider their decision before applying. Many students who graduate from master's degree programs should anticipate entering a limited job market and be aware of the fact that most doctoral programs prefer accepting students with a bachelor's degree.

The status of master's-level psychologists has been debated ever since the doctorate was established as the standard for full member status in the APA. The main reason for this policy was to ensure insurance coverage for clinical psychologists. It was feared that psychology would lose stature with insurance carriers and government agencies if it were to accept the master's degree as sufficient for private practice.

The student considering a master's-level program should not be naive about the ethical standards of educators. Educators make a living by selling their wares. The student-consumer must exercise the same caution employed when buying an expensive product or service. Thus, learn whether the degree in question will open doors to employment by discussing prospects with professionals in local clinics, hospitals, and schools. Find out how they view the degree under consideration.

The Bachelor's-Level Psychologist

During the 1970s, an outpouring of government funds created many new jobs in the mental health field. Persons with two- and four-year college degrees were sought after by agencies and clinics. This lush phase is definitely behind us. The current job market offers few opportunities for B.A.-level people.

There are occasional openings for psychometrists to administer and score certain tests or for psychiatric aides in hospitals. According to a 1991 survey by the Bureau of Labor Statistics, approximately one-quarter of the estimated 70,000 students who graduated as psychology majors, with a B.A. degree, were able to find employment. Typically, they were able to secure positions within the mental health field, entailing:

- conducting intake interviews at crisis intervention centers;
- being case managers for the elderly or people with disabilities; or
- working as counselors in halfway houses, prisons, and psychiatric hospitals.

LICENSING AND CERTIFICATION

The American Board of Professional Psychology (ABPP) examines psychologists in clinical, counseling, and school psychology. The examination for the clinical specialty is based on a written report submitted by the candidate as well as on the direct observation of the candidate in a clinical encounter with an actual patient. Once the candidate fulfills these requirement, he or she is awarded the prestigious status of diplomat.

Of more importance than ABPP diplomas are the certificates and licenses awarded by the various states. Two types of state laws have been enacted. A certification law restricts the use of the title psychologist to someone who has met prescribed standards. Some states require a Ph.D. or Psy.D. for certification, and almost all demand satisfactory performance on an examination. Certification laws do not in any way regulate the practice of psychotherapy. In many states, virtually anyone can offer services as a psychotherapist, counselor, or hypnotherapist without any legal restrictions.

The other type of law confers a license as a psychologist. A license defines a profession in terms of its function as well as ethical and professional standards. Only a licensing law could prevent unqualified people from practicing therapy. Unfortunately, most of the state laws now are merely certification laws. Employers generally require certification for higher-level positions in clinical psychology.

SALARIES

As in other professions, salaries depend on education, degree, setting, experience, and number of work activities. Graduate students begin to earn some money during the internship; salaries are modest, ranging from $12,000 to $15,000 per year. The intern is not expected to be fully productive and receives valuable training and experience that make up for the low salary. The Veterans Administration, for example, continues to be a major contributor to the training of clinical psychologists. Students are paid and are not obligated to continue with the VA after training.

Beginning salaries for the doctoral psychologist range from about $37,000 to $44,000 per year in the private sector. According to a 1995 survey by the American Psychological Association, the median salary for a clinical psychologist with a Ph.D. and a minimum of five years experience is $51,000 per year in a clinic or public hospital. These jobs are generally competitive and difficult to get. The beginning professional with limited or no experience is therefore encouraged to seek employment in a less competitive market. Usually, federal agencies (such as the VA) will offer good salaries and are receptive to hiring the starting psychologist. The VA begins fully trained psychologists at Federal Grade 11, which has a starting salary of $36,609. The VA notes that 80 percent of its professional psychologists are at Federal Grade 13. The starting salary for this Grade is $52,176. In 1997, the average salary for psychologists in the federal government in nonsupervisory, supervisory, and managerial positions was about $62,120 a year.

The psychologist who chooses to work at a college or university will receive a lower starting salary than in a clinical setting. However, clinical jobs usually demand an eleven-month, thirty-five-hour a week schedule, whereas academic jobs call for nine or ten months with a twelve- to fifteen-hour teaching schedule. Psychologists who teach are paid on the basis of professional rank in the same way as specialists in other fields. Beginning salaries for assistant professors range from about $32,000 to $36,000 per year. Those who reach the higher ranks of associate and full professor can expect to earn substantial salaries. Again, salaries vary depending on the college or university.

ABD psychologists are generally paid less then those with doctorates, receiving salaries generally proportional to the amount of completed education. In 1995, the annual median salary for a master's-level psychologist was $38,000 in counseling psychology and $41,000 in clinical psychology.

Certified doctoral psychologists have the option of adding to income by going into private practice. The average fee for psychotherapy with a clinical psychologist is $90 per session, with considerable variation.

JOB DESCRIPTIONS

Here are some typical job listings provided by government agencies.

Title: Clinical psychologist internship
Location: A medical center in a New England city
Salary: $12,000 per annum

Qualifications: The applicant must be enrolled in an APA-approved clinical or counseling doctoral program.

Duties: The intern will rotate in outpatient, inpatient, and day treatment services. The program calls for closely supervised training in psychological testing, and in individual, group, and family therapy. Opportunities are available to work in substance abuse.

Title: Forensic psychologist
Location: A college of criminal justice
Salary: Commensurate with academic rank
Qualifications: Substantial experience as a psychologist in a police, family court, or correctional setting. Some teaching experience required.
Duties: Teach courses in a master's program in forensic psychology.

Title: School psychologist
Location: A country school system
Salary: $45,000
Qualifications: The applicant must have a master's degree in psychology. Some experience as a school psychologist is desirable. Must be certified as a school psychologist.
Duties: Duties include administration of standardized tests as well as consulting with parents and teachers about student problems. Travel within country required.

Title: Assistant professor of community psychology
Location: Department of Psychology in small college
Salary range: $32,000 to $34,000
Qualification: Ph.D. in clinical or community psychology.
Duties: The candidate will teach introductory courses in community psychology, supervise students in external placements, and advise students.

Title: Senior clinical psychologist
Location: An outpatient child guidance clinic
Salary range: $50,000 to $55,000
Qualifications: The applicant must have a Ph.D. in clinical psychology, state certification, plus several years of postdoctoral experience.
Duties: The principal duties are to provide group, marital, and family therapy to families or referred children. The candidate must also supervise interns in an APA-approved program.

Title: Chief psychologist
Location: Comprehensive community mental health center

Salary range: $54,000 to $61,000

Qualifications: Ph.D. in clinical psychology, state certification, and postdoctoral experience.

Duties: Position involves coordination of psychiatrists and social workers, program evaluation, and supervision of psychology trainees.

PROFESSIONAL ORGANIZATIONS

American Psychological Association
Research Office and Education in Psychology
Accreditation Offices
750 First St. N.E.
Washington, D.C. 20002
www.apa.org/

American Psychological Association
P.O. Box 2710
Hyattsville, MD 20784-0710
(800)374-2721

Educational Psychology Home Page
www.apap.org/divisions/div15

REFERENCES

American Psychological Association. (1996). *Psychology/careers for the twenty-first century: Scientific problem solvers.* Washington, D.C.: Author.

Appleby, D. (1997). *The handbook of psychology.* Reading, MA: Longman.

Cass, J., & Birnbaum, M. (Updated frequently). *Counselor's comparative guide to American colleges.* New York: Harper & Row.

Clay, R. (1997). *Two states move closer to gaining Rx privileges.* Washington, D.C.: American Psychological Association.

DeGalan, J., & Lambert, S. (1995). *Great jobs for psychology majors.* Lincolnwood, IL: VGM Career Horizons.

Garfield, S. L. (1974). *Clinical psychology: The study of personality and behavior.* Chicago: Aldine.

Murray, B. (1997). *Learning to be stewards of community well-being.* Washington, D.C.: American Psychological Association.

Phares, J. E. (1984). *Clinical psychology: Concepts, methods, and profession* (rev. ed.). Homewood, IL: Dorsey.

Rheingold, H. (1994). *The psychologist's guide to an academic career.* Washington, D.C.: American Psychological Association.

Spaver, A. (1976). *Career choices in psychology.* New York: Messnew.

Super, C. M., & Super, D. E. (1994). *Opportunities in psychological careers.* Lincolnwood, IL: VGM Career Horizons.

U.S. Department of Labor, Bureau of Labor Statistics. (1998–1999). *Occupational outlook handbook.* www.stats/bls.gov/oco/ocos060.htm

Woods, P. J., & Wilkinson, C. S. (1987). *Is psychology the major for you? Planning for your undergraduate years.* Washington, D.C.: American Psychological Association.

SOURCES OF ADDITIONAL INFORMATION

Newsletters

- *The Clinical Psychologist*
- *The Counseling Psychologist*
- *Division 17 Newsletter* (counseling psychology)
- *The Industrial-Organizational Psychologist*
- *Newsletter for Educational Psychologists*
- *The School Psychologist*

Journals

- *Clinical Psychology: Science and Practice*
- *Educational Psychologist*
- *School Psychology Quarterly*

CAREERS IN PSYCHIATRY

WHAT IS PSYCHIATRY?

Psychiatry is the medical specialty devoted to the diagnosis and treatment of emotional, mental, and behavioral disorders, including such problems as substance abuse. Patients helped by psychiatrists suffer from a variety of psychological disorders, ranging in severity from mild to incapacitating. In addition to treatment, psychiatrists study the causes of psychological disorders and try to find ways of preventing as well as relieving them.

WHY CHOOSE PSYCHIATRY?

Like other branches of medicine, psychiatry is extremely rewarding—in many respects, not simply financially. A career as a psychiatrist offers an opportunity to help others, relieve human suffering, and perhaps find new methods of treating—even curing—psychological disorders. And in addition to high prestige and substantial income, psychiatry offers opportunities for leadership. Psychiatrists are needed and aggressively recruited in rural areas, in public hospitals, and in primary care settings.

DEVELOPMENT OF PSYCHIATRY—CAREER TRENDS

Psychiatry as a medical specialty dates back to the mid-1800s. In those days, psychiatrists devoted themselves largely to the care and treatment of the mentally ill in hospital settings. "Mental" disorders were thought to be due to physical defect caused by specific abnormalities of the brain and nervous system. This emphasis on brain function accounts, at least in part, for the traditional association of psychiatry with neurology, the study of the nervous system and the brain. However, as an example of how a field may come full circle, in the same century that psychiatry had once emphasized psychological models, it has now turned again to functions of the brain and tends to deemphasize psychotherapy.

At the beginning of the twentieth century, psychiatrists turned away from neurology to psychology, to psychoanalysis in particular. Psychiatrists joined others in the helping professions who had begun to recognize that certain "mental" disorders, called *neuroses,* were caused not by physical but by psychological factors. Sigmund Freud, founder of psychoanalysis, advanced the idea that neurotic symptoms were caused by ideas and impulses that are beyond conscious awareness. Freud evolved a complex theory of personality now considered one of the great achievements of recent history. Under Freud's leadership, psychoanalysis became a powerful social and intellectual movement.

Alfred Adler and Carl Jung, once closely associated with Freud, broke away from him and founded rival movements of their own. Adler taught that neurotic symptoms were caused by the need to compensate for feelings of inferiority. Jung believed that the psychological problems of modern men and women were often due to the neglect of religious and spiritual needs.

A second generation of psychoanalytic thinkers, including Harry Stack Sullivan, Karen Horney, and Erich Fromm, extended analytic thinking to include cultural and family influences on behavior. The influence of the psychoanalytic movement reached its zenith during the 1940s and 1950s, when it was particularly fashionable in the United States. Young psychiatrists increasingly sought training in psychoanalytic institutes.

The wave of enthusiasm for psychoanalysis crested in the late 1950s. Then, predictably, a backlash set in. Psychoanalytic therapy was criticized on the grounds that it was costly, ineffective, and overly long. The basic idea was that neurotic symptoms would be relieved if certain unconscious memories and ideas were uncovered during the treatment. In many cases, this uncovering process seemed to drag on for years. Also, because the method called for three to five sessions a week, it was obvious that only wealthy clients could afford treatment. A psychoanalyst might have only four or five patients in treatment at any one time. During the turbulent 1960s, psychoanalysis was criticized by social reformers on grounds that it was irrelevant to the needs of the poor and disadvantaged.

Psychiatrists were accused of abandoning the mentally ill in hospitals and of devoting too much time to the care of a small number of wealthy neurotics, most of whom might function without psychiatric help. As criticism mounted, the percentage of medical school graduates who chose psychiatry as a specialty declined. Meanwhile, there was a veritable explosion of new therapies. Literally hundreds of new therapies have been developed within the past three decades, many opposed to traditional psychiatric methods. Psychiatry seemed to be under attack from every quarter.

It is difficult to predict the future of such a turbulent field, though in view of opportunities for pathbreaking research and treatment, "dynamic" rather than "turbulent" may be a more accurate characterization. The trend seems to be toward a return to the traditional focus on serious mental disorders. Many psychiatrists are particularly interested in research on the biochemical basis of serious mental illnesses. Psychiatrists are moving away from psychoanalysis and emphasizing those treatments in which they can make best use of their medical training.

Admittedly, a "physician surplus" in the United States has developed during the 1990s. The Council on Graduate Medical Education reports an oversupply of specialist physicians (and psychiatry *is* a specialty) and an undersupply of primary care doctors such as family physicians or pediatricians. However, it is not really clear whether the United States has too many or too few psychiatrists.

Ultimately, the determination of how many psychiatrists the United States needs will derive from decisions about what *kinds* of care will be provided to individuals experiencing psychological troubles and—equally important—*who* will provide that care. For example, some troubled people will need medications such as tranquilizers as part of their care. These medications must be prescribed by a physician, but does the physician have to be a psychiatrist? The answer will influence the size of the workforce in this specialty. Or, to what extent will psychiatrists provide psychotherapy for their patients as well as monitoring their prescription medications? The question of supply and demand for a profession is very complex and made even more so by social change, including managed care, and new developments in research and treatment that change the psychiatrist's role and the way psychiatric care is delivered.

Two factors suggest that the number of medical students choosing psychiatry will rise during the first decade of the twenty-first century. First, many health specialties are crowded, and new graduates are likely to take a second look at psychiatry and other fields that offer better than average employment opportunities. Second, new resources to support the work of psychiatrists have contributed to renewed public respect for the field. As an example, 20 years ago the excessive use of shock therapy, in the minds of some authorities, contributed to negative views of the field. Yet, in 1985 a federal advisory panel cautiously endorsed carefully conducted electroshock treatment for special groups of patients, especially those suffering from depression.

You can get a further sense of the range and complexity of psychiatric research, treatment, and current trends by sampling recent journals, in print or cyberspace. Most of the professional organizations listed at the close of this chapter, such as the American Association for Medical Education or the American Psychiatric Association, have their own Web pages. A number of the over 124 medical school departments of psychiatry also publish in cyberspace. These resources include, for example, Psychiatry Hotlinks from Johns Hopkins and the University of Michigan's Psychiatry Star. Osteopathic medical schools are also included; they grant the D.O. rather than the M.D. degree to their graduating physicians.

WHAT DOES THE PSYCHIATRIST DO?

The majority of psychiatrists devote part of their professional time to treating patients, which is obvious because the great majority maintain a private practice. On the other hand, few psychiatrists devote all of their working hours to treatment. The average psychiatrist puts in about 50 hours a week, dividing this time between hospital or clinic work, consultations, supervision, and private practice. Psychiatrists also teach, conduct research, and perform administrative duties. We will review their major activities, beginning with treatment.

Psychiatric Treatment

In general medical practice, there is usually a close connection between diagnosis and treatment. The doctor examines the patient in an effort to arrive at a correct diagnosis. The diagnosis (meaning the nature of the disorder) determines the treatment in a very direct way. For example, if the patient is diabetic, the doctor may prescribe a certain diet along with insulin treatment. In psychiatric practice, the relation between diagnosis and treatment is not as clear. The patient is usually attempting to cope with a very complex stress situation. To understand the patient's symptoms, the psychiatrist takes into account the patient's family life, financial resources, education, and work status. Once a comprehensive picture is formed, the psychiatrist selects one or a combination of treatments. The choice ranges from medication to shock therapy to various forms of psychotherapy. All psychotherapies involve verbal communication in the context of a relationship between doctor and patient.

As previously described, until the 1950s, most psychotherapists used psychoanalytic methods. During the next decade there was a rapid, almost explosive, development of new therapies. Some of these were little more than popular rehashings of Freud's ideas. Others represented serious attempts to apply humanistic concepts to therapy. For example, existential, client-centered, and gestalt therapies all emphasize the uniqueness and capacity for growth inherent in the human being. The humanistic therapist does not play the role of expert but relates to the client on an equal basis. The therapist helps the client accept full responsibility for his or her choices in life.

A quite different approach to therapy, called *behavior modification,* is based on learning and conditioning theories. Behaviorists reject the idea that mental patients' behavior is of a different kind than that of normal people. They assume that all behavior is learned and potentially capable of being unlearned. Mental patients are seen as people who have learned ways of behaving that are inconvenient or socially undesirable. Behaviorists also devised programs that significantly improve the behavior of mental patients in hospitals. The basic approach is simply to "reinforce" desirable behavior such as active participation in a ward meeting by means of some reward that the client finds gratifying.

Originally, most psychotherapy was conducted on a one-to-one basis. During the 1920s and 1930s, only a few therapists practiced *group therapy.* Today, group methods are widely used by psychiatrists, psychologists, and social workers. The techniques range from supportive treatment to a kind of group psychoanalysis. Groups may be employed for almost any problem, from weight reduction to marital discord. Group differs from individual therapy in that there is usually less emphasis on uncovering deep-seated conflicts and more on present-day relationships with other people.

The group usually consists of eight to twelve clients meeting with the therapist on a weekly basis. The members may share some common problem such as career difficulties, marital unhappiness, or child-raising conflicts. Other groups include persons with varied problems; each member may simply be trying to find ways of improving his or her relationships with others. The therapist encourages the members to share their feelings and experiences with each other. Group therapy is not simply a watered-down form of individual therapy. A cohesive group with an effective leader can exert a powerful influence on each member to change behavior in constructive ways.

Medical Therapies

Psychotherapy is only one form of treatment that the psychiatrist may employ. As a medical doctor, the psychiatrist can also use medication or even shock therapy to change a patient's mood, feelings, or behavior. Neither of these treatments can be used by nonmedical therapists.

Shock therapies were originally developed to treat schizophrenia and other forms of serious mental illness. There are several kinds, all of which involve the deliberate induction of temporary convulsions in the patient. Over the years, various drugs and procedures were employed to induce seizures, sometimes with disastrous results. It was eventually found that the safest and most convenient means of inducing shock was ECT, electroconvulsive shock therapy, which involves passing an electric current across the frontal lobes of the brain. The current is applied by electrodes placed at the patient's temples. The shock, which lasts only a fraction of a second, causes the patient to convulse and lose consciousness. It is now generally accepted that ECT is not particularly help-ful to schizophrenics but may be effective against severe depression, and this is its major present-day use. The use of ECT has been branded as barbaric by some critics, partly on the grounds that it destroys—at least temporarily—some short-term memory.

Doctors have prescribed herbs and medicines for emotional ills since the beginning of recorded history. It was only in comparatively recent years that researchers found ways to isolate the active chemicals in traditional remedies. These modern techniques led to the development of *psychopharmacology*, the study of drugs that can change a person's mood or outlook on life. These are also called *psychoactive drugs*.

The introduction of potent tranquilizers in the 1950s revolutionized the treatment of serious mental disorders. In correct dosage, these drugs reduced anxiety without making the patient dull or sleepy. With the aid of these drugs, many patients were able to leave the mental hospital and live in the commu-nity. In some cases, the medication was helpful in making patients more receptive to psychotherapy.

Medication is still a major form of treatment for seriously disturbed patients. These drugs do not produce a cure of psychotic states but simply help reduce the severity of acute symptoms and make the patient more manage-able. Patients who stop taking the drugs are subject to recurrent psychotic episodes.

During recent years, many other types of psychoactive drugs have been developed. For example, antidepressants such as Prozac or Zoloft help ele-vate the mood of depressed patients. Lithium is often helpful to patients who are subject to extreme mood swings (bipolar mood disorders).

The Psychiatrist As Leader

Aside from direct treatment of patients, the psychiatrist's other duties vary depending on the nature of the setting in which he or she is employed. The psychiatrist who runs a hospital or a large clinic spends little or no time in treat-ing patients but serves as an administrator whose main function is to provide the framework within which clinicians do their work. The administrator plans the budget, raises funds, establishes policies, and hires and fires personnel. This work requires a combination of clinical experience and a flair for man-agement. The importance of high-level administration can hardly be overesti-mated. A failure at this level can have disastrous consequences for the entire hospital. Capable administrators are always in short supply and are, therefore, able to command relatively high salaries.

A psychiatrist working in a mental hospital is generally the leader of a treatment unit, which may be a ward or unit of the hospital. Psychiatry is one of the few fields in which a recent graduate can begin as team captain. The traditional mental health team consists of the psychiatrist, a psychologist, and a social worker. The team discusses such matters as treatment, discharge of improved patients, and ward routine. Input from nurses, aides, and various therapists is taken into account. In recent years, psychologists and social workers have been challenging the notion that the team leader must be a psychiatrist.

The larger the number of patients in the unit, the less likely that the psychiatrist will be able to devote much time to direct contact with patients. Some psychiatrists feel frustrated about the amount of time they must devote to paperwork, administrative duties, and medical management (that is, monitoring patients' psychoactive drug regimens). Regrettably, psychiatrists are given little training in administration, although they are required to do a significant amount of it.

Psychiatric Consultation

Consulting is the process of giving expert advice or testimony about some matter relevant to mental health. Psychiatrists act as consultants to the courts, prisons, schools, and other agencies. The psychiatrist who works in a general hospital is a consultant to other medical specialists. For example, the psychiatrist may be asked to examine a surgical patient who has become violent for no apparent reason. In another case, the psychiatrist may be asked to counsel a patient about a lifestyle that contributes to physical illness.

Research

Because the profession brings important knowledge and insight to research problems and because its members can make important contributions to the field, the scarcity of funding for large-scale research is sometimes a source of frustration. Research is costly and opportunities are often dependent on the federal government and private foundations. Lean periods alternate with rich periods.

The range of possible research topics is immense. The psychiatrist may study the effect of a new drug on depression, the impact of certain patterns of mothering on children's development, or the ways in which people react to the stress of unemployment. Aside from such major projects, the psychiatrist often spends a certain portion of his or her time in informal research studying the literature about a certain disorder or writing up an unusual case for publication in a psychiatric journal.

Community Psychiatry

This is a relatively new approach to psychiatry based on the assumption that the community must assume responsibility for the mentally ill. It is no longer acceptable to shunt mental patients into hospitals far from the neighborhoods in which they once lived. The main goals are to prevent mental illness by means of community programs and to help mental patients fit into the community. A psychiatrist working in this area is often associated with a community mental health center. He or she might devote time to setting up residences for former mental patients or to arranging programs for them. In addition, the community psychiatrist helps coordinate local efforts to maintain a healthy social environment. For example, the principal of a school may want advice about dealing with racial tensions among the students. The mayor of the town might want to discuss the possibility of an after-school program for teenagers. Setting up programs for senior citizens might also call for some input from the community psychiatrist. This is an exciting and challenging career experience for the person who enjoys community development.

A Day in the Life of a Psychiatrist

A graduate of a medical school in Louisiana, Jorge is a psychiatrist with many years of clinical experience. He is the founder and director of a private family therapy agency. The agency, located in downtown Philadelphia, has three main purposes: to treat disturbed families, to train students in family therapy, and to conduct research. These varied purposes are reflected in the following account of a typical busy day in Jorge's professional life.

9:00–9:45 A.M.: The first hour at the agency is reserved for looking at the mail, making telephone calls, and generally getting organized. In response to a letter, Jorge dictates a response accepting an invitation to deliver a keynote address at a regional mental health conference.

10:00 A.M.–1:00 P.M.: Intake meeting. Present are two senior staff members, one a psychologist and the other a social worker. The purpose of the meeting is to decide what to do about 15 new families applying for outpatient treatment. The staff decide that eight of the families would be suitable for student therapists. However, the other families are assigned to more experienced staff members because of the potential for suicide and substance abuse problems of some family members.

1:10–1:45 P.M.: Jorge interviews a prospective candidate for the job of video technician. This is an important job because many therapy sessions are videotaped and used for training purposes.

1:00–2:00 P.M.: After lunch, Jorge conducts a regular seminar in family therapy for first-year students. He discusses some basic principles of marital counseling, using videotapes and case material from his own practice.

2:10–3:00 P.M.: Chart review and medical management. Jorge checks several patients who have been coming to the agency for several months and receiving regular doses of psychoactive drugs. He reviews their lab results and speaks for about 15 minutes with each one.

3:15–4:00 P.M.: He meets with a senior staff member to discuss the details of a research project of a new FDA-approved antidepressant drug and its use with persons displaying multiple substance abuse patterns.

4:10–5:00 P.M.: Jorge consults with a staff therapist about several families that are not responding favorably to treatment.

In general, Jorge enjoys the varied activities that heading an agency requires of him. The only cloud on the horizon is that Jorge and other senior staff psychiatrists find themselves doing less and less psychotherapy with patients and spending more of their time prescribing psychoactive drugs. Jorge and his colleagues think that the drugs are effective and have few side effects. However, they worry about "compliance": the drugs will work only if the patients take them. The most troubled patients, with whom Jorge would like to spend more time, are often the least likely to take their drugs exactly as prescribed.

How Does One Become a Psychiatrist?

Preparation can begin as early as the high school years. Ideally, the student should enroll in a first-rate academic or college preparatory program. In particular, the student should demonstrate an aptitude for science and mathematics. It is also helpful to establish a record of being a well-rounded person by participating in extracurricular activities. If a premedical club, such as the Future Physicians Club, is available, the student should definitely join. Working in a hospital or laboratory as a volunteer is fine, but this could wait until the college years.

It cannot be emphasized too strongly that the student needs to master good study habits. Many students who sail through high school have trouble with college work. Learning to comprehend textbook material, studying for exams in a consistent way, and taking good lecture notes are some critical skills. The struggle to get into medical school is fiercely competitive, and a poor student is soon eliminated.

Selecting a College

The first step is to find out about the academic standards of the colleges under consideration. Try to get information about the number of candidates who are accepted into medical school from each college. Obviously, the college must offer those courses that are prerequisites for admission to medical school. Your premedical program should include courses in both general (inorganic) and organic chemistry, biology, physics, and English. Look into the quality of the faculty, especially the science instructors. Does the faculty have a good reputation? Do they have doctoral degrees? If possible, visit the college and talk to students, counselors, and teachers. If there is a premedical adviser, certainly speak with that person, too.

Applying to Medical School

Medical schools employ several criteria in deciding which candidates are accepted. One criterion is college grades, particularly in science courses. The great majority of serious applicants have at least a B+ average. Because grading policies vary among schools, medical schools also take into account Medical College Admission Tests (MCAT) scores, which provide a standard way of comparing applicants. An MCAT score of 30+ is usually required for acceptance at a medical school. Admission committees also consider recommendations from faculty members at applicants' colleges. These letters can be particularly important for a student who is borderline in grades or MCAT score.

Some outstanding candidates apply for early admission—that is, after three years of college. If interested, ask about the early admissions program when you contact medical schools. It is unwise to apply for this unless you are very confident of your academic ability. It is rare for a medical school to accept an applicant below the age of twenty.

You may apply to medical school in several ways. The centralized application approach for schools awarding the M.D. degree is through the American Medical College Application Service (AMCAS). The advantage of this approach is that you need fill out only one AMCAS application, and a copy of your consolidated application is sent to all AMCAS schools to which you are applying. As of 1997, you can even file your application on-line. Further information about this service may be obtained from your premedical adviser or by contacting the AMCAS, in care of the American Association of American Medical Colleges (AAMC), Section for Student Services. Osteopathic medical schools offer a similar on-line application process through American Association of Colleges of Osteopathic Medicine Application Service (AACO-MAS). (See "Professional Organizations.") Other useful applicant publications from the AAMC include the *Medical School Admission Requirements* (updated and published annually).

Your other option is to apply directly to each medical school of your choice. You should apply during the summer of the year preceding your enrollment. Make sure your application material is typed and neat. Answer all questions. A transcript and recommendation must go to each school to which you are applying directly.

There is much discussion on college campuses today about how hard it is to get into medical school. Actually, being accepted by a medical school is competitive but not impossible; about one-third of all applicants are accepted, although not necessarily by their first-choice school. The number of medical schools has increased over the past few decades, as have medical school departments of psychiatry in the United States, which numbered 124 in the mid-1990s.

Medical School

Medical school is an intense and demanding four years of study. The first years emphasize normal biology including anatomy, biochemistry, and physiology. The class time is about evenly divided between lectures and laboratory procedures. Clinical demonstrations are often included in lectures so that the subject matter is related to real patients. All medical schools in the United States have basic courses in psychiatry that are required of all candidates regardless of future plans to specialize.

During the third year, the student becomes familiar with the practical techniques of diagnosis. Formal lectures on surgery, pediatrics, and other specialties are supplemented by case histories. Students are assigned patients for a "work-up," which includes a physical examination and an interview concerning the patient's medical history. The student makes a preliminary diagnosis on the basis of the data gathered and determines what laboratory tests are needed. Needless to say, a faculty member supervises all aspects of the student's work. The student rotates among various departments and becomes familiar with a wide variety of illnesses. The trainee gradually assumes the status of a real doctor, participating in ward rounds and conferences. The practice of medicine with real patients does not begin all at once but proceeds in a gradual, step-by-step fashion.

During the fourth year, called the *clerkship*, still more responsibility is assumed by the student who may be on call 24 hours a day and *must* be ready to assist in emergencies. The trainee receives the M.D. degree after the completion of four years of training. However, for the prospective psychiatrist there is still a long road ahead.

Residency

The psychiatrist-to-be now undertakes four years of advanced training. The initial year may include study of internal medicine, family practice, or pediatrics. The subsequent three years are devoted to intensive training in psychiatry. The training may take place in an accredited psychiatric hospital, the psychiatric department of a general hospital, or a university medical center. The American Psychiatric Association supervises the quality of the training. The psychiatrist-to-be gains experience with patients of various types and of all ages.

A typical training program would include courses in clinical psychiatry, personality development, psychopathology, history of psychiatry, child and adolescent psychiatry, psychosomatic medicine, and psychotherapy. However, these formal courses are only one aspect of the work. Even more important is direct contact with patients. At this stage of training, the doctor is responsible for the treatment of patients, sometimes on an individual basis. Typically, the resident is rotated from service to service within the hospital. The resident may begin training on a ward for adult inpatients and then after a year be switched to a child or adolescent service. The trainee is closely supervised by a staff psychiatrist. It should be noted that the typical first-year resident salary is at least $30,000.

Osteopathic Medical Schools

Graduates earn a doctor of osteopathy (D.O.) degree, are licensed to perform surgery and prescribe medicine, and are eligible to apply to residency programs in psychiatry and other specialty areas of medicine.

Foreign Medical Schools

Many applicants rejected by U.S. medical schools could have done well in medical training. One option for the rejected applicant is to pursue a career in some related health area. Another possibility is to seek admission to a foreign (usually called international) medical school, even though the educational standards are not usually as high as those in U.S. medical schools. Thousands of American students are attending medical schools in Mexico, the Philippines, Italy, Belgium, Spain, and the Caribbean. Most of these students plan to return to the United States to practice or to continue their medical training. *Barron's Guide to Foreign Medical Schools* is a useful publication in this area, and the Educational Commission for Foreign Medical Graduates helps set standards for certification of doctors who did their training overseas.

Tuition

Because tuition costs at medical schools have been rising steadily, it is difficult to provide exact information. In the late 1990s, the average annual cost for first-year students at private U.S. medical schools was between $25,000 and $30,000 for tuition and fees only; these figures do not include living expenses.

At public (state-sponsored) medical schools, average tuition and fees approached $10,000 per year for state residents and almost double that for nonresidents. Other expenses, including books, supplies, and room and board might cost an additional $10,000 to $12,000.

Loans and Scholarships

The student should not be discouraged by the high costs of medical education. The fact is that over 80 percent of medical students borrow money to cover their expenses. Furthermore, a variety of grants and loans are available. Information can be obtained from the AMA and the AAMC (see "Professional Organizations"). Two very useful AAMC publications are *Financial Planning and Management for U.S. Medical Students* and *Minority Student Opportunities in United States Medical Schools.* The federal government and the armed forces also support medical education. Another good source of up-to-date information about grants, loans, and scholarships is the catalog of the medical school(s) to which you plan to apply.

CERTIFICATION

Even after satisfactory completion of the residency, the doctor is not yet awarded a diploma in his specialty. The American Board of Psychiatry and Neurology is responsible for certifying the competence of psychiatrists. The board issues certificates in (1) psychiatry, (2) neurology, (3) child psychiatry, and (4) child neurology. The applicant for a diploma in either psychiatry or neurology must have completed three years in residency approved by the Council on Medical Education of the American Medical Association and have had two full years of satisfactory work experience. A list of approved training programs is available from the American Medical Association (see "Professional Organizations").

Psychiatrists who wish to specialize in child psychiatry generally complete a two-year training program in a children's psychiatric hospital or clinic *after* completing the training in adult psychiatry. Before taking the examination for the diploma in child psychiatry, the candidate must already have a diploma in general psychiatry.

The examinations for each specialty include both written and oral parts. Usually, basic information about the field is covered in the written part, whereas the oral part includes the examination of patients under supervision of an examiner. Board certification is not a legal requirement for the practice of a specialty. However, the doctor who has earned his or her diploma enjoys the full acceptance of the medical community. This acceptance may sometimes be translated into practical benefits such as job offers from prestigious institutions.

SALARIES

The salaries of psychiatrists vary widely depending on seniority, experience, the kind of work, and setting. The lowest salaries are usually offered by the state mental hospitals, which is one reason they fail to attract enough qualified psychiatrists. Other settings such as community health centers or private hospitals pay considerably higher salaries. During the mid-1990s, the average annual salary of a staff psychiatrist in a clinic or hospital setting was $110,000. Administrative positions generally pay more than staff positions.

However, salaries are only one source of income for psychiatrists. As mentioned earlier, almost all psychiatrists maintain a private practice in addition to their salaried job. The fee for a private session with a psychiatrist currently ranges from $115 to $250 per nominal hour session. After expenses are deducted, the median (midpoint) income from all sources for psychiatrists averaged about $120,000 per year in the mid-1990s. Moreover, the psychiatrist can increase income by working more hours.

In psychiatry, as in all other fields, income and supply and demand are closely linked. In the 1960s, between 7 and 10 percent of the graduates of U.S. medical schools went on to specialize in psychiatry. In the early 1980s, that figure had dropped to only about 4 percent. In the 1990s, half the residencies in psychiatry were filled by graduates of international medical schools.

JOB DESCRIPTIONS

A good way to learn about career opportunities in psychiatry is by looking at job offerings. These can be found in some psychiatric journals as well as in newspapers of large cities. Here is a selection of typical job offerings adapted from actual advertisements.

> **Title:** Forensic psychiatrist
> **Location:** The Department of Psychiatry of an eastern university
> **Salary range:** $60,000 to $75,000 per annum
> **Qualifications:** This is a postresidency fellowship for one year with an opportunity for faculty appointment. The candidate must have completed an approved residency training program.
> **Duties:** The duties include giving expert testimony in court and providing consultations within the following forensic settings: a maximum security prison, prosecutor's office, and public defender's office. The

candidate will also assist a university-based research team investigating long-term effects of maternal use of crack cocaine among incarcerated offspring.

Title: Child and adolescent psychiatrist
Location: Tertiary hospital in the Midwest
Salary: $115,000 plus incentives and benefits
Qualifications: Board certified.
Duties: Join hospital staff of two adult psychiatrists' comprehensive services from partial programs, in-home services, covering inpatient units (including a 14-bed detox unit). Majority of work is outpatient in very modern facilities. Opportunity for faculty appointment at medical school.

Title: Director of community mental health services
Location: State Department of Mental Health of a midwestern state
Salary range: $75,000 to $100,000
Qualifications: Completion of residency plus two years of postresidency experience. In addition, the candidate must have at least one year of experience in a high-level administrative post.
Duties: This is an administrative position that involves directing a countywide program of mental health services including facilities for mental retardation, alcohol and substance abuse, and outpatient mental health; responsibilities include coordinating the activities of satellite clinics.

Title: Child psychiatrist
Location: A county mental health center in a western state
Salary range: $81,000 to $90,000
Qualifications: ABPN certification in child psychiatry. Candidate must be able to work with a multidisciplinary team and a variety of referral sources.
Duties: The position involves diagnostic evaluations, treatment consultation, psychotherapy, and medication therapy of children and adolescents.

Title: Child and adolescent psychiatrist
Location: Hospital in a southwestern state
Salary range: $80,000 to $100,000
Qualifications: Several years of experience beyond residency with demonstrated administrative skills.
Duties: A high-level administrative post that will involve designing a new division of the hospital for seriously disturbed youngsters. Duties will include establishing intake policies and procedures, setting up

liaison with schools and other community agencies, planning treatment approaches, and staffing.

PROFESSIONAL ORGANIZATIONS

American Academy of Child and Adolescent Psychiatry
3615 Wisconsin Ave. N.W.
Washington, D.C. 20016
(202) 966-7300
www.aacap.org

American Association of Colleges of Osteopathic Medicine
5550 Friendship Blvd., Suite 310
Chevy Chase, MD 20815-7231
(301) 968-4100
www.aacom.org

American Medical Association
51 N. State St.
Chicago, IL 60610
(312) 464-5000
www.ama-assn.org

American Psychiatric Association
1400 K St. N.W.
Washington, D.C. 20005
(202) 682-6000
www.psych.org

Association of American Medical Colleges
2450 N St. N.W.
Washington, D.C. 20037-1126
(202) 828-0400
www.aamc.org

Educational Commission for Foreign Medical Graduates
3624 Market St., 4th floor
Philadelphia, PA 19104-2695
(215) 386-5900
www.ecfmg.org

REFERENCES

Alexander, F. G., & Selesnick, S. T. (1995). *The history of psychiatry: An evaluation of psychiatric thought and practice from prehistoric times to the present.* New York: Harper & Row.

Sales, B. D., & Shuman, D. (Eds.). (1996). *Law, mental health, and mental disorder.* Pacific Grove, CA: Brooks/Cole.

Schmolling, P., Youkeles, M., & Burger, W. (1997). *Human services in contemporary America* (4th ed). Pacific Grove, CA: Brooks/Cole.

Sen, N., & Sparrow, I. (Eds.). (1997). *The complete guide to foreign medical schools: In plain English.* Wayland, NY: Indus.

Wright, J. W. (1996). *The American almanac of jobs and salaries* (serial). New York: Aaron.

CAREERS IN THERAPEUTIC RECREATION

WHAT IS THERAPEUTIC RECREATION?

According to the National Therapeutic Recreation Society:

> Leisure and recreation are human rights and are critical to human health and well-being. People with disabilities or limitations may require assistance in using their leisure to enhance their physical, social, emotional, intellectual and spiritual abilities. This principle applies equally to people who live in communities and to those who require short- or long-term clinical or residential care. Services are delivered through a continuum of care—therapy, leisure, education, and recreation participation—in order to enable and empower people to develop and maintain health, well-being, and appropriate leisure lifestyles. (www. RecreationTherapy.com)

Therapeutic recreation uses recreation activities as a form of treatment to serve the ill and disabled. The individual may be physically disabled, mentally challenged, and/or have serious social problems. Whereas recreation is engaged in for enjoyment, therapeutic recreation focuses on corrective or rehabilitative goals in addition to pleasure. If a disability is permanent, the recreation therapist would help the disabled person accept his or her disability and live and work as fully as possible within its limitations. If the limitation is a temporary one, the individual would be helped to regain the former level of functioning. Even though recreation is therapeutic when used as a form of treatment, recreation cannot and does not actually cure a disease or eliminate a disability.

WHY CHOOSE THERAPEUTIC RECREATION?

People usually choose a career in which they hope to gain satisfaction and enjoyment. Therapeutic recreation provides abundant opportunities for attaining these benefits. It meets the desire to help others and also provides the additional pleasure of engaging in recreational activities. Therapeutic recreation is a growing field, and the increased recognition of its importance has created a need for additional trained personnel and enhanced its acceptance by many health professionals. The job outlook is quite good, and opportunities exist throughout the country, with steadily rising salaries.

DEVELOPMENT OF THERAPEUTIC RECREATION—CAREER TRENDS

The development of therapeutic recreation must be seen in relation to the development of the recreation profession. The broader recreation field includes national, state, and city parks and recreation departments, community center programs, and other programs that provide leisure-time activities. This movement arose in the last half of the 1800s. At the same time, a growing number of hospitals, institutions serving the mentally challenged, and mental institutions began providing recreation activities to their patients. However, these efforts were limited in scope. The importance of the contribution that recreation makes to the ill and disabled was not really recognized until World War I, when recreation was discovered to play a significant part in treating disabilities and shortening the length of hospitalization.

The relationship between recreation and rehabilitation was confirmed in the 1920s and 1930s. During that period, there was an organized effort to establish departments of recreation within institutional settings. In addition, the use of recreation personnel in veterans' institutions expanded. After World War II, a more intense push was made to the development of recreation programs and services for the ill and disabled. The sudden and widespread growth of institutions serving the armed forces and veterans resulted in a need for large numbers of recreation workers. At the same time, the need for recreation programs and services in private hospitals and other institutions increased along with the population in these facilities.

In 1949, the Hospital Recreation Section of the American Recreation Society was formed. Three years later the National Association of Recreation Therapists was created. The National Recreation and Park Association was formed in 1965. One year later, the National Therapeutic Recreation Society was established as a member of that parent organization. The merger of the various groups spurred surveys and research to determine recreation needs. It was determined that there were well over 25 million individuals in need of therapeutic recreation services in 1965, and today the number is increasing. Many colleges and universities are training therapeutic recreation specialists in an attempt to meet this need.

WHAT DOES THE RECREATION THERAPIST DO?

Recreational therapists work as members of an interdisciplinary team often consisting of a physician, psychologist, social worker, and nurse. As a member of such a team, the recreation therapist has several duties and responsibilities. Initially, when a recreation therapist is assigned a client, he or she will collect relevant information from several different sources: medical records, medical staff, and family members. The recreational therapist will then assess the client's strengths and weakness and develop a treatment plan based on the client's needs, abilities, and interests. The client then will be encouraged to participate in an activity or activities that the recreation therapist feels will be useful and therapeutic. The ultimate goal for the recreation therapist is to plan and develop individualized activities or interventions that help the client remediate the effects of an illness or disability and improve physical, cognitive, and social functioning.

The recreation specialist can provide three levels of direct service. The first level is centered on providing activities for rehabilitation purposes. The goal is to use activities to help raise the functioning level of a person who has physical, emotional, or social disabilities. The therapeutic recreation specialist controls and directs the activity with the emphasis on attaining therapeutic goals. The recreation therapist may, for example, prescribe an assertiveness program to help a depressed client achieve greater self-confidence and independence. In other cases, the recreation therapist may encourage a client to attend a music activity as a way of encouraging socialization with other clients and adjustment in a new facility.

The second level of direct service is to help the disabled individual see and use recreative activities as a form of enjoyment. The recreation therapist and the disabled individual plan the program together. The therapist helps the person learn skills and knowledge so that he or she may eventually become self-directed in meeting his or her leisure needs.

The third level of direct service is with those disabled and ill people who are able to enjoy and participate in recreational activities on their own. The recreation therapist in this case provides recreation facilities, programs, and opportunities for the individual.

In all three levels of service, the recreation therapist can work with individuals or groups depending on the need of the participants. In the institutional or treatment setting, the emphasis of recreation programs is more toward rehabilitation than education or recreation. In nontreatment facilities, the reverse is generally true.

Nontreatment facilities include parks, settlement houses, YMCAs, senior centers, community centers, and recreation centers. The programs provided in these facilities for the disabled are referred to as "recreation for special populations." As indicated previously, the primary focus in nontreatment facilities is on education for leisure and recreation for special populations. Although most therapeutic recreation specialists work in treatment settings, the need for trained specialists in the community is great and continues to grow. Many professionals, in addition to recreation specialists, now believe that individuals leaving treatment facilities would benefit greatly if recreation services were more available in their communities. Although we are seeing some growth in this area, additional training and financing by the government and private agencies are still needed.

One area that has received some attention during the last decade is the role of the recreation therapist in our schools. Recently, administrators, teachers, parents, and counselors have been using recreational therapy in their quest to meet student needs. The recreation therapist will often make important and relevant suggestions designed to help students with issues such as socialization, vocational training, and developing healthy leisure activities. Recent research strongly suggests that by using recreational activities in our school systems, students can develop a positive self-image and learn to interact with others in a meaningful and constructive way.

The following sections discuss in more detail some of the different roles and opportunities available to the person interested in pursuing a career in therapeutic recreation.

Supervision

Supervision has two basic purposes. First, it is a method of helping a less experienced recreation therapist learn from an experienced professional. The transmission of knowledge and skills is the essence of this work. Second, supervision ensures the effectiveness of the beginning professional. It is also used to provide support to the staff and make sure that the service provided is in line with the policies and directives of the administrator.

In addition to supervising a staff of professionals and volunteers, the role of the supervisor also includes writing policy, designing and implementing new interventions, consulting and interacting with other specialists, and developing relationships with outside community agencies.

Consultation

This area of therapeutic recreation service focuses on helping other professionals become more effective in their work. Because it is very difficult to keep up with the rapid growth of knowledge, skills, needs, and pressures, the recreation therapist must use outside help to ensure provision of the most effective service. The consulting recreational specialist might give suggestions and advice regarding new approaches for staff training or program development. Because of increasing needs for new programs, the need for consultants is also increasing.

Research

Research is a rapidly expanding area of therapeutic recreation, with the primary focus on developing new approaches and techniques. For example, is it more effective to make participation in activities mandatory or optional? Is it helpful to know the life history of a disabled person to devise a specific therapeutic program? Research is also essential in determining the recreation needs of disabled people in a community or society. If the needs can be predicted or identified, the recreation specialist can better plan to meet those needs.

Research is also a form of evaluation used to determine whether a service is accomplishing what it should. If not, why not, and how might it be improved? Or should the service be dropped and the funds used elsewhere?

Education

Recreation education is one of the many specialties essential to the development and transmission of new theories, knowledge, information, skills, values, and ethics of the profession. The primary function of the educator is the training of recreation therapists. The educator must be knowledgeable not only in therapeutic recreation but also in closely related fields such as occupational therapy, activities therapy, dance therapy, and social work. Educators must be in constant contact with what is happening in the institutions and communities with regard to practical problems, changing conditions, and new approaches so that they might use that knowledge in their teaching and training.

Another aspect of education in which every recreation educator or recreation therapist should be actively involved is educating laypeople and professionals about the importance of therapeutic recreation services for the ill and disabled. Such enhanced understanding of the recreational therapist's role will only further enhance the field's recognition and acceptance as a vital human service.

A Day in the Life of a Recreation Therapist

Florence earned her bachelor's and master's degrees in therapeutic recreation at an eastern university. She is presently employed as the director of recreational therapy in a large nursing home serving over 100 older adults. Many of the residents are disabled in some way and are, therefore, limited in their ability to take part in recreational activities. For example, some have heart conditions, and many suffer from arthritis. Some use wheelchairs, and others are withdrawn, isolated, and depressed.

A typical day for Florence in the nursing home might look like this:

8:00–9:00 A.M.: Florence meets with a physician, social worker, nurse, and physical therapist to discuss treatment plans for the residents. Florence makes recommendations regarding activities that will help the residents enjoy themselves and promote health and vitality. The activities also help residents develop skills that increase their level of functioning and self-image.

9:15–10:00 A.M.: Florence works with a group of residents confined to wheelchairs. She helps them learn how to play charades while confined to the wheelchairs. Learning different ways of using their bodies while enjoying themselves, such as bending over to pick up objects or twisting their bodies to act out the name of a dance, not only helps the participants gain satisfaction and a desire to participate in other activities but increases their level of functioning and thereby promotes a more positive self-image.

10:15–10:30 A.M.: Florence writes her report on the group. She notes each resident's progress during the activity with regard to enjoyment, willingness to participate, enhancing skills, relationships, and self-esteem.

10:45–11:30 A.M.: Florence works with a retired schoolteacher who is depressed and who isolates herself from other patients and most staff. Florence, through the use of puzzles of various kinds, (for example, crossword, jigsaw), attempts to help her enjoy herself, generate an interest in activities that are intellectually stimulating and challenging, and relate to other residents who enjoy such stimulation and challenge. Her patient showed interest in working with the puzzles but refused to have anything to do with other residents. She also showed some movement, and Florence will continue to encourage her to relate to other residents.

11:30 A.M.–12:00 P.M.: Florence writes up her notes on the individual patient to present at a team meeting the following morning.

1:00–2:00 P.M.: Florence visits residents in their rooms to discuss the kinds of activities they would like to participate in during future sessions. She also discusses changes shown by the residents during activities and encourages them to continue participation.

2:00–2:30 P.M.: As part of her administrative responsibilities, Florence makes arrangements for facilities, equipment, and supplies needed for upcoming activity sessions with various groups and individuals.

2:30–3:00 P.M.: As part of her supervisory responsibilities, Florence visits and observes the various activities being conducted by her staff. She is concerned about a staff member planning an all-day trip.

3:00–3:30 P.M.: Florence meets with the director of the home to discuss budget, staff, program, equipment, and other issues for which she is responsible. She raises the problem of limited equipment available for her program and the need for a half-time worker to meet the growing needs of the residents.

3:30–4:00 P.M.: Florence meets with one of her staff in a supervisory conference to discuss the problems the therapist had in helping the group plan the all-day trip.

Florence's duties and responsibilities, entailing direct practice, supervision, and administration keep Florence interested and challenged. She looks forward to her work even though she is often frustrated when residents do not respond to her and her staff's efforts.

How Does One Become a Recreation Therapist?

The minimum requirements for becoming a professional in therapeutic recreation is an associate's degree from an accredited college with a major or emphasis in therapeutic recreation. Students with an interest in becoming a therapeutic recreation specialist should pursue a baccalaureate degree in therapeutic recreation. A master's degree in therapeutic recreation is yet another way of entering the ranks of professional recreation therapists. At present, over 150 colleges and universities offer therapeutic recreation programs at the undergraduate level, and over 50 provide graduate programs.

Although not mandatory, some volunteer or paid work while in school with organizations, institutions, or agencies that provide recreation services would be helpful. If the student can gain experience working in a recreation program serving physically and emotionally disabled individuals, so much the better. Also, the student should learn activity and recreation skills, including games, sports, dance, or arts and crafts.

At the college level, typical therapeutic recreation courses include Leisure Activities for Special Populations, the History and Development of Therapeutic Recreation, Principles and Practices of Therapeutic Recreation, Organization of a Recreation Program, and Recreation for the Aging and Mentally Challenged. In addition to courses in recreation and therapeutic recreation, courses in biology, psychology, sociology, and physical education are helpful, as are public speaking, physiology, and writing courses.

Some programs break down the therapeutic recreation courses based on specific disabilities. For example, at least one program provides courses in Therapeutic Recreation with the Developmentally Disabled, Therapeutic Recreation with the Physically Handicapped and Aged, and Therapeutic Recreation with the Emotionally and Socially Disabled.

Almost all programs include internships or fieldwork under the supervision of an experienced recreation specialist. The field experience should involve working with physically and/or emotionally disabled individuals. The extent or length of time of the internship varies from college to college but is usually required for two semesters. Therapeutic recreation programs at the master's level might well include courses in Administration of Therapeutic Recreation Services, Consultation in Therapeutic Recreation, advanced courses in Recreation for the Ill and Disabled, and Recreation Services for the Ill and Disabled. Advanced internships on this level are usually mandatory and require the student to devote a minimum of 360 hours under the supervision of a certified therapeutic recreation specialist.

Programs vary from one institution to another. Therefore, try to get as much information as possible on the different programs to make the choice that best meets your needs and interests. See "Professional Organizations" for a list of groups providing this information.

LICENSING AND CERTIFICATION

A program of voluntary registration for therapeutic recreation specialists is offered through the National Council for Therapeutic Recreation Certification (NCTRC; see "Professional Organizations"). Presently, certification is not mandatory; however, many jobs do strongly suggest that candidates for recreation positions possess certification (that is, as a certified therapeutic recreation specialist, or CTRS). Students interested in obtaining certification should contact the NCTRC for up-to-date requirements.

The purpose of certification is to help gain recognition for qualified recreation therapists as professionals. In 1991 the American Therapeutic Recreation Association published *Standards for the Practice of Therapeutic Recreation,* which have helped improve the status of the therapeutic recreational specialist within the health care profession.

Presently, there is no common regulatory procedure for this profession. Each state has its own set of licensure, certification, or regulation of titles standards, so it is up to the prospective therapist to learn what these standards are for his or her respective state.

SALARIES

The beginning average salary for a therapeutic recreation specialist with a baccalaureate degree in therapeutic recreation is $33,000. The average annual salary for administrators, consultants, and supervisors is about $42,000. Students with a two-year associate's degree in recreational therapy can anticipate earning an annual salary of $22,000. Salaries vary from state to state and may also depend on what type of agency the therapist decides to work in. For example, the annual average salary in the federal government for nonsupervisory, supervisory, and managerial positions is about $39,400.

Job responsibilities also affect the amount one may earn at the beginning level as well as at higher job levels. The following section's examples of typical job announcements obtained from newspapers, government announcements, and journals will provide a clearer picture of what kind of opportunities are available.

JOB DESCRIPTIONS

Title: Recreation special programs coordinator (therapeutic recreation)
Location: Midwestern city's recreation department
Salary range: $33,266 to $36,005 annually
Qualification: CTRS
Duties: Employee has total responsibility for planning, developing, promoting, coordinating, supervising, and evaluating city wide TR programs. Responsible for hiring, training, supervising, and evaluating assigned staff for specific tasks, activities, and programs.

Title: Recreation therapist II
Location: State hospital
Salary: $23,876 (part-time, twenty hours per week)
Qualifications: B.A. degree from an accredited college or university. One year's experience as a recreation therapist or a master's degree in therapeutic recreation from an accredited college or university may substitute for experience. Must be eligible for certification as a CTRS by the NCTRC.
Duties: Provide comprehensive therapeutic recreation services to assigned caseload; evaluation of patients and documentation of services. Must be flexible regarding working schedule, as late afternoon, evening, and weekend services are provided for our clients.

Title: Recreation therapist
Location: Special Olympics
Salary: $33,456 per year
Qualifications: Bachelor's degree in therapeutic recreation plus three years' experience in a community setting. Current CPR/first aid competency is required. CTRS certification is preferred.
Duties: Community outreach and relations, supervision of part-time and seasonal staff, recruitment and training of volunteers, safety and risk management, program administration and budgeting, and other duties as assigned.

Title: Therapeutic recreation specialist
Location: 120-bed subacute rehabilitation hospital
Salary: Competitive salary and full benefits package
Qualifications: Bachelor's degree in therapeutic recreation; CTRS preferred.
Duties: Organizing, planning, and running therapeutic recreation groups. Responsible for individual patients, attending team meetings, and documentation.

Title: Activities therapist
Location: Private nursing home
Salary range: $22,000 to $27,000
Qualification: Associate's degree in therapeutic recreation.
Duties: Assist senior staff members in the planning and implementation of various recreation activities. Some interviewing and documentation of patients' progress.

PROFESSIONAL ORGANIZATIONS

American Therapeutic Recreation Association
P.O. Box 15215
Hattiesburg, MS 39402-5215
www.atra-tr.org

National Council for Therapeutic Recreation Certification
P.O. Box 479
Thiels, NY 10984-0479

National Therapeutic Recreation Society
22377 Belmont Ridge Rd.
Ashburn, VA 20148
www.nrpa.org/branches/htrs.htm
E-mail: NATRSNRPA@aol.com

References

Austin, D. (1996). *Therapeutic recreation: An introduction.* Boston: Allyn & Bacon.

Compton, D. (1997). *Issues in therapeutic recreation: Toward the new millennium.* Champaign, IL: Sagamore.

Cordes, K. A., & Hilmi, I. (1996). *Applications in recreation and leisure for today and the future.* New York: McGraw-Hill.

Frye, V., & Peters, M. (1972). *Therapeutic recreation: Its theory, philosophy, and practice.* Harrisburg, PA: Stackpole.

Gunn, S. L., & Peterson, C. A. (1978). *Therapeutic recreation program design, principles and procedures.* Upper Saddle River, NJ: Prentice Hall.

Kelley, J. D., et al. (1977). *Therapeutic recreation educator: Guidelines for a competency-based entry-level curriculum.* Alexandria, VA: National Recreation and Park Association.

Kisner, C. C., & Aleen, L. (1996). *Therapeutic exercise: Foundations and techniques.* Philadelphia: Davis.

Kraus, R. (1983). *Therapeutic recreation service, principles, and practices* (2nd ed.). Philadelphia: Saunders College.

MacLean, J. (Ed.). (1983). *Aging and leisure.* Alexandria, VA: National Recreation and Park Association.

Mosey, A. C. (1973). *Activities therapy.* New York: Raven.

O'Morro, G. S. (1980). *Therapeutic recreation: A helping profession.* Reston, VA: Reston.

Sources of Additional Information

Journals and Newsletters

- *Creating Solutions* (P.O. Box 28223, San Diego, CA 92198-0223; [619] 277-6337)
- *Creative Forecast* (P.O. Box 7789, Colorado Springs, CO 80933-7789; [719] 633-3174)
- *Preparing for a Career in Therapeutic Recreation* (National Recreation and Park Association)

CAREERS IN ART THERAPY

WHAT IS ART THERAPY?

One definition of art therapy is "the purposeful use of art to meet and express psychological needs." A former president of the American Art Therapy Association (AATA) has defined it as "the use of art and artistic processes specifically selected and administered by an art therapist to accomplish the restoration, maintenance, or improvement of the mental, emotional or social functioning of an . . . individual."

Art therapy does not focus on the development of the aesthetic capabilities of clients but rather on their ability to use and manipulate a variety of visual media to create images and thus communicate thoughts and feelings. Often, the disciplines of art and therapy are combined as a therapeutic tool and, equally important, as a diagnostic tool as well. Through observation and analysis of art behaviors, art products, and the client's nonverbal and verbal communications, the art therapist formulates a diagnostic assessment and treatment plan as part of a total therapy program. Art therapy may be used as a primary therapy or as an adjunct to other forms of psychological and physiological therapy. For those who are mentally or emotionally ill or who are physically challenged, art therapy provides access to the inner workings of the mind through the assessment of visual expressions rather than just verbal expressions.

WHY CHOOSE ART THERAPY?

A career in art therapy provides a unique opportunity for an individual to combine training in the visual arts with human services. The art therapist may work with a group of other professionals in an institutional setting and develop a private practice as well. It is a viable choice for the aesthetically creative individual because it allows the professional to remain in contact with the manipulation of various visual media, while at the same time deriving a great deal of satisfaction from helping people understand their problems and function better.

Art therapists may practice with individuals, groups, and/or families in many settings. Art therapists have become increasingly more accepted in the process of diagnosis, assessment, and treatment and serve to lead the activities of groups of clients toward greater self-expression and self-understanding. Professional advancement usually involves supervising and coordinating other professionals, administering expressive therapy programs, and/or teaching.

The field of art therapy has given rise to the development of professional organizations such as the AATA and the Society for the Arts in Healthcare, the latter being a coalition of 22 institutions (including outstanding medical facilities) that believe that art in its varied forms can humanize the health care environment and help people open their minds and emotions to healing. The interest in the field has resulted in an increase of published works regarding techniques and case studies. Professional journals, such as the *American Journal of Art Therapy* and *Design for Arts in Education* are also gaining in popularity and professional acceptance within the field of human services. It is fairly common to find job vacancy announcements regarding art therapists in most major newspapers.

Art therapy is a growing occupation as a result of hospitals, schools, and nursing homes recognizing the value of creative arts as preventive and remedial therapies. There will likely be a dramatic increase in the percentage of art therapists employed in treating the elderly over the next twenty years because this population will grow substantially. According to the Career Information Center, the outlook for employment is very good through the year 2005. The essential qualifications for an effective art therapist include an understanding of art media, strong interpersonal skills, patience, emotional stability, creativity and spontaneity, and insight into human psychological processes.

DEVELOPMENT OF ART THERAPY—CAREER TRENDS

Since the early 1800s, societal concern for the mentally ill created a context in which the creative arts could be considered as useful in treatment. In the first years of the twentieth century, a recognition developed that the making of art was important in the rehabilitation and maintenance of a patient's mental health. Later, in the 1930s, several works were published on creativity and artists by respected scholars and therapists. At this time, staff at the Menninger Clinic recognized that the arts provided health benefits to their patients and began to employ artists, dancers, musicians, and writers.

Not until the late 1940s, however, were there specific books pertaining to the theory and technique of art therapy. One of the leading pioneers in the field, Margaret Naumburg, introduced theories concerning the therapeutic use of graphic expression. She emphasized the basic approach of using art as a tool for psychotherapy. In fact, the roots and formation of the field of art therapy were strongly influenced by Freud's psychoanalytic theories. As research with individuals expanded, Naumburg uncovered methods of using art as a primary therapeutic method rather than an additional tool for the trained psychotherapist. In the 1950s, techniques were developed for using art in working with adolescent boys in residential treatment centers. In 1958, art was introduced into the evaluation and treatment techniques employed by the National Institute of Mental Health.

In 1961, the *Bulletin of Art Therapy* was begun as a means of educating, stimulating, and supporting colleagues in the field; it was later renamed the *American Journal of Art Therapy*. In 1964, the first Creative Arts Therapies Department was developed within a mental health facility at the Division of Social and Community Psychiatry at Albert Einstein College of Medicine in New York City. The arts therapies were integrated into clinical intervention and research. They were part of an interdisciplinary approach within a psychiatric setting using the concept that nonverbal media can directly tap into the emotional rather than the cognitive processes of the patients. In addition, it provided certain patients with a visible and tangible link to reality and the present.

For some 20 years after the first publications of material on art therapy, many attempts were made at organizing a professional, national organization of art therapists. In 1968 a series of lectures hosted by Hahnemann Medical College in Philadelphia provided the stimulus to finally develop guidelines to establish such a group, which culminated in the founding of the AATA in 1969. The formation of this organization provided a professional identity for art therapists and helped develop standards and criteria pertaining to professional training. Since then, the amount of literature devoted to art therapy has increased. The *American Journal of Art Therapy* has become the professional journal in the field. In 1969, two graduate programs leading to a master's degree in art therapy were initiated. Today, approximately 25 offer master's programs and two, a doctorate. Specific clinical facilities now offer art therapy training programs as well as providing for supervised work experience.

The development of managed health care systems has become increasingly more important as the number of creative arts therapists has grown in institutionalized settings. Their effect on how the institutions and individual practitioners make decisions regarding the services provided, the length and degree of treatment, and the amount of freedom and autonomy on the job will be significant in the years ahead.

What Does the Art Therapist Do?

The art therapist often functions as a member of a therapeutic team that might include a psychologist, psychiatrist, and social worker. Other specialists, such as a music therapist or dance/movement therapist, could be added to this team as dictated by the needs of the patient as well as the resources and personnel available.

Art therapy is often quite effective as a tool in treatment and diagnosis. Often patients can become so involved and absorbed in their creative endeavors that their psychological defense mechanisms, which would have previously prevented them from functioning at a healthier level, become more relaxed and therefore more visible and accessible to the therapist.

Art therapists work with people of all ages who may suffer from varying degrees of psychological and/or physical impairment. Such a population might include individuals with psychological problems ranging from the mildly disturbed to the severely psychotic. Another group might encompass persons suffering from physical and/or disease-related disorders, such as stroke, mental impairment, or the loss of a limb. However, art therapists are not limited to working with an impaired or disabled population. It is becoming increasingly common now for art therapists to work with populations within traditional school settings and personal growth centers, because healthier individuals may derive therapeutic benefits from artistic expression as well. It is important to understand that the individual is not judged on artistic abilities, nor is previous art experience necessary.

The value of artistic expression is in the process of creation. This process is sometimes referred to as a form of "symbolic speech." A form of communication is developed between client and therapist through visual images. It becomes the art therapist's role to help the client identify and integrate what these expressions mean. In art therapy the stress is not to produce a meaningful product but rather to develop an atmosphere of acceptance and interest without judgment or criticism.

The artwork alone does not provide the totality of diagnostic tools, however. In observing and discussing the client's creative activities, the therapist considers the client's past history, records, existing visual language, the content of staff conferences, as well as the medium used; the organization of the work; its size, form, color, lines, focus, motion, detail, content, affect, texture, and mass; and the actual story that the client is able to verbalize, if possible. Such information as the client's choice of colors and materials often provide meaningful insights for the therapist that help in both diagnosis and treatment. In addition to various other functions previously discussed, the art therapist works as a guide to the art materials available to the client. The therapist must have a thorough knowledge of how to use a variety of different media such as pastels, watercolors, charcoals, clay, oils, and acrylics and be able to teach the techniques for using these materials.

There are several approaches to art therapy. One approach views art as an adjunct to traditional psychotherapy. The actual creation itself—the choice of colors or the form—expresses elements of the person's unconscious as well as certain personality traits. By using art in this manner, people can freely express aspects of themselves that they can or will not express verbally. This point is clear when working with young children's artwork, for example. In working with children, the art therapist should offer a variety of pleasurable, visual stimuli that encourage responses and sustained attention. As they work, children often become verbal and talk about what they are doing as it unfolds, thereby providing insight into the thought processes. In a group setting, children may even eventually begin to talk among themselves and possibly share materials or collaborate on a project. In this way children can see themselves in relationship to others with the accompanying roles and communication.

Art therapy may also be used as a therapy by itself. Art, or the creative process, is seen as the therapeutic means of resolving emotional conflicts, developing personal growth and self-awareness, and providing a direct outlet for self-expression. Here, the therapist is mainly concerned with the individual's inner feelings and experiences and how these feelings become apparent when expressed through the creative process. There are many examples of the creative process becoming a form of therapy. More and more frequently, for instance, a businessperson may seek relief from the day's tensions by working creatively with clay, sculpting a piece of marble, or painting a picture. For the emotionally troubled person, this means of self-expression can release stored-up feelings that may otherwise be expressed in a destructive manner. Communicating very personal ideas and feelings through art can lead to the achievement of a sense of well-being and satisfaction.

Art therapists most commonly work within a group setting with anywhere from three to ten clients at a time. They may work with individuals and families. As described earlier for children, within a group, the various art creations themselves can serve as a vehicle for interaction among the group members. The therapist can function as a facilitator for group discussions concerning the individual art expressions. In this context, people who have difficulty expressing themselves verbally to other individuals can find art a suitable vehicle for such expression.

Art therapy as practiced with families provides similar benefits. In this setting, the art therapist can help the family learn to communicate more clearly with one another. A typical therapy technique is to ask all members of the family to draw pictures of one another or to draw a house, a tree, and a person. It is during the discussion of the drawings afterward that the art therapist can help the family members identify any discrepancies or distortions in how they see themselves, how other family members see them, and how they would like to be viewed.

Depending on the particular situation and the available materials, the art therapist can use several other techniques. Clients are often instructed in the use of clay and are then given a small block of clay that needs to be pounded, slapped, kneaded, and hit with their hands and/or a mallet, before shaping it into an object.

Another technique involves providing an assortment of cut-out figures, portraits, interior scenes, landscapes, and objects (these materials are gathered from magazines prior to the group's meeting) for clients to combine into a collage that expresses a personal portrait of their lives and has symbolic significance. Sometimes, on a very large sheet of paper (size is dependent on the group's size) clients are asked to communally create a mural with the theme of an upcoming season or holiday.

Usually crayons, pencils, or paints are available for the clients' use to create images by free-associating their dreams, wishes, or hopes for the future. An interesting practice is using a scribbling technique in which clients are asked to draw a line without premeditating what they are doing and keep the point in contact with the paper at all times, using pencil, colored pencil, pastels, or charcoal. When viewed afterward, the spontaneity of the line may suggest an object, person, animal, or pattern that the client can then embellish or modify.

The art therapist works with older people in settings such as nursing homes, hospitals, psychiatric and rehabilitation facilities, senior centers, and day treatment programs. The value of art therapy here is not just as a treatment for the infirm or institutionalized person but also as a valuable tool in the prevention of illness and the maintenance and promotion of health through rediscovery of oneself, enhanced interaction and communication, increased confidence, life review, a sense of new meaning, and improved decision-making skills.

Within general and psychiatric hospitals, art therapy departments are growing. Art therapists work directly with clients as well as offer training courses to other hospital personnel in the techniques and concepts of art therapy. Many art therapists are actively involved in research projects within the hospital setting. Art therapists may serve as consultants to a public or private school interested in incorporating art therapy into a curriculum. Some innovative programs have been initiated establishing art therapy in prisons and working with the terminally ill in institutional settings. Art therapists can be found working within institutions for the emotionally disturbed, learning disabled, hearing or visually impaired, and physically challenged. They also work with individuals who are in severe physical pain, with the homeless in shelters, with individuals in bereavement groups, and with war veterans and refugees who are attempting to deal with the effects of posttraumatic stress disorder.

Art therapists also serve in university counseling clinics, and as the field develops, there will be an increase in art therapists teaching in art therapy programs within colleges and universities. Some art therapists also function as consultants in many public and private settings.

Treatment is either short- or long-term and may vary in frequency depending on particular needs—usually one hour for individuals and one-and-a-half to two hours for groups. The space in which art therapy takes place should be adequate in terms of size, location, lighting, storage, furnishings, and flexibility. Materials and methods must be simple and easy, able to be controlled by the clients, easily cleaned up, colorful, and conducive to large motor activity. The art therapist often maintains and repairs the art materials and equipment as well.

A Day in the Life of an Art Therapist

Judy is a professional art therapist who works full-time in the psychiatric unit of a large public hospital in a major urban area of the United States. This is a residential facility, and Judy works on the locked ward in which are housed seriously disturbed mental clients. Judy possesses a B.F.A. degree in illustration with a minor in art therapy, as well as a master's degree in graphic design and poetry. In addition, she completed one year of coursework in art therapy. The combination of training in fine arts and an extensive internship at the undergraduate level helped earn her AATA certification over 20 years ago. A typical day for Judy is as follows:

8:30–9:00 A.M.: Judy selects the art supplies and other materials for the day's program and is sure to have enough materials so that all the clients can have the same items to avoid competition or anxiety.

9:00–10:00 A.M.: Judy meets with the first group of clients (12) in a large open room with tables to work on. She is accompanied by an attendant at all times. During the session she presents a theme to the group about which each client is encouraged to draw. This is designed to elicit individual responses to topics that are emotionally stimulating.

10:00–11:00 A.M.: Judy conducts another group session with a similar number of clients in which they are encouraged to work with clay.

11:00 A.M.–Noon: Judy participates in a team meeting with other professional staff, including a medical doctor, psychiatrist, social worker, and nurse. They discuss the individual cases and various modes of treatment and are kept abreast of client observations and behavior.

Noon–1:00 P.M.: Lunch in the hospital cafeteria.

1:00–2:00 P.M.: Judy conducts another group session in which the clients work with colored pencils.

2:00–3:00 P.M.: Judy conducts another group session in which the clients work with water-based paints.

3:00–4:30 P.M.: Judy meets with the psychiatrists and presents her clients' work. She provides her thoughts and interpretations in each case, as well as her observations of the clients concerning their actual behavior while they were doing the work.

Judy enjoys her work a great deal and feels that she has been adequately prepared through her academic, artistic, and practicum training. This profession permits her to combine her skills, interests, and genuine concern for people, as well as her ability to encourage creativity using a variety of media often accompanied by music. She occasionally works with a music therapist, which adds another dimension to a job that encourages alternative modes of self-expression for individuals who have great difficulty communicating verbally or in writing.

How Does One Become an Art Therapist?

The AATA has established specific criteria for educational preparation and training in art therapy. According to the AATA, to be recognized as a professional art therapist, one must obtain a master's degree or complete clinical training in an institute or clinic. After all training is completed, one can apply for registration with the Art Therapy Credentials Board (ATCB) to become a board-certified registered art therapist (ATR-BC). Therefore, graduate-level education and/or training is considered to be the minimum for an entry-level position in the field. Programs providing for education and training in the field are still a relatively recent development. In considering the training as an artist and a therapist, the practitioner should be able to conduct research in the field and be a skilled writer as well. One must complete the required core curriculum as outlined in the AATA Educational Standards to qualify as a professional art therapist. Entry into the profession is now at the master's level, requiring either one of the master's degrees described earlier or 21 graduate credits in art therapy with a master's degree in a related field.

The necessary positive personal qualities of a successful art therapist are caring and concern for others, self-awareness, openness, intelligence and intuition, inventiveness and creativity, empathy and the ability to draw on negative personal experiences, articulateness, and the social skills and ability to inspire confidence. It is also important that much of art therapy training be experiential to develop personal professional self-awareness.

Undergraduate Preparation

At present, people wishing to pursue a career in art therapy must first attend an accredited undergraduate academic institution. Undergraduate students must concentrate in the basic areas of fine arts and the behavioral and social sciences. The AATA advises "strong preparation in these two areas, in addition to a good general background in the humanities, as the basis for specialized Art Therapy training in accordance with the Association's standards." During the undergraduate period, those interested in pursuing graduate-level training in art therapy should first attempt to work as volunteers in agencies or institutions serving a variety of populations. Firsthand experience is one of the best ways of determining one's own suitability to this field.

Graduate Preparation

Graduate study in art therapy is required, and most schools require at least two years of study in art therapy. Graduate education includes both coursework and fieldwork.

The curriculum includes such courses as the history of art therapy, techniques, practical applications to selected populations, and psychological diagnostic and evaluation methods. In supervised fieldwork, sometimes referred to as field training or the practicum, the student is placed in an institution or agency that encourages creative expression. The student is closely supervised by a faculty member representing the graduate program. During this period of time, usually a minimum of 600 hours in the field or two full academic semesters, art therapy techniques become refined. In addition, the student is encouraged to personally undergo the experience of the art therapy. This further develops personal skills and provides a means for obtaining additional insights into the art therapy experience.

Upon completing graduate school, the student is awarded a master's degree. Some are called master's of science in art education, master's of arts in art therapy, master's of arts in art, and master's of creative arts in therapy.

In addition to academic programs, art therapists also attend specialized institutes and clinical programs that offer certificates of completion. Often, institutes and clinical programs provide opportunities to pursue further training in specialized areas within art therapy (for example, techniques for working with specific populations such as children, the elderly, or the physically challenged).

LICENSING AND CERTIFICATION

There now exists the Art Therapy Credentials Board (ATCB), which, as an independent organization, grants postgraduate registration (ATR, a registered art therapist), upon review of documented completion of graduate education and postgraduate supervised experience. The registered art therapist who successfully completes a written examination administered by the ATCB is considered board certified and must maintain the credential through the accumulation of continuing education credits.

The ATCB reviews the academic and training credentials of those who wish to sit for a written examination leading to board certification as a registered art therapist (ATR-BC). The board requires an additional 1,000 hours of direct supervised clinical experience beyond the 600 hours of practicum required for the master's degree. In certain places of employment a different form of credential may be needed, such as public schools requiring that an art therapist be licensed as a teacher before being able to function as an art therapist.

As previously mentioned, the AATA has worked toward establishing standards for the training and preparation of art therapists. Registering with AATA signifies that a minimum level of proficiency has been attained.

SALARIES

Typical starting salaries for art therapists range from $19,000 to $25,000 per year depending on the quality of educational background, experience, type of institution, and geographic location. In states listing art therapist in their job classifications, regular salary increments can be expected. The median income is $28,000 to $38,000 per year, with the top earning potential for salaried administrators running between $40,000 and $60,000 per year. Art therapists in private practice constitute a much smaller percentage of art therapists than those employed within hospitals, institutions, and agencies. Payment for private individual art therapy sessions ranges from $75 to $90 per hour for those with a doctorate. The individual sessions usually last from one to one-and-a-half hours, usually meeting once a week. It is not at all uncommon for experienced art therapists to pursue the doctoral degree in a related field with the intent of teaching at the university level in programs designed to train art therapists. Salaries for such individuals employed full-time at the university level can be approximately $50,000 per year.

JOB DESCRIPTIONS

The following represent a selected sample of job descriptions for art therapists found in newspapers, journals, and professional newsletters.

Title: Staff art therapist
Location: Large midwestern psychiatric institution
Salary range: $19,000 to $23,000 per annum
Qualifications: Minimum of three years' experience working in a similar setting with the older adult population. Must possess a master's in the field and be ATR-BC.
Duties: To function as a member of a treatment team with psychiatrist and social worker. Direct client contact with individuals in group settings. Must have the ability to keep accurate records.

Title: Instructor or assistant professor of art therapy
Location: Small college in New England
Salary range: $28,000 to $35,000 per annum
Qualifications: Minimum of five years' experience in the field, functioning in a variety of clinical or rehabilitative settings. Must have prior teaching experience, preferably at the college or university level. Must be ATR-BC. Master's degree required, doctorate preferred.
Duties: Teach within expressive therapies program. Must be able to teach introductory and advanced courses as well as supervise art therapy students in field placements.

Title: Director of Art Therapy Department
Location: Large psychiatric hospital on the West Coast
Salary range: $37,000 to $42,000 per annum
Qualifications: Minimum of six years' experience working within similar settings. Three years' experience as supervisor or program director. Master's required. Must be ATR-BC.
Duties: To supervise an expanding art therapy program. Responsible for budget allocation, supplies acquisition, and supervision of staff of three full-time therapists. Some evening and weekend work will be required.

PROFESSIONAL ORGANIZATIONS

American Art Therapy Association
1202 Allanson Road
Mundelein, IL 60060-3808
(847) 949-6064
www.arttherapy.org

Art Therapy Credentials Board, Inc.
401 N. Michigan Ave.
Chicago, IL 60611
(312) 527-6764

REFERENCES

Agell, G. (1997, November). Art therapy literature and managed care. *American Journal of Art Therapy, 36,* 46–48.

AJN Newsline. (1995, July). *American Journal of Nursing, 95,* 65, 67.

American Art Therapy Association Publications. (1996, 1997). [Assorted titles; write 1202 Allanson Road, Mundelein, IL 60060-3808.]

Ault, R. (1992, June 19). Aging artfully: Health benefits of art and dance. *Testimony before the U.S. Senate Special Committee on Aging.* Washington, D.C.: U.S. Government Printing Office.

Burroughs, H., & Kastner, M. (1993). *Alternative healing* (pp. 21–23). La Mesa, CA: Halcyon.

Carlisle, J., & Donald, K. M. (1985, October). The use of art exercises in assertiveness training. *Journal of Counseling and Development, 64*(2), 149–150.

Feen-Calligan, H., & Sands-Goldstein, M. (1996, November). A picture of our beginnings. *American Journal of Art Therapy, 35,* 43–59.

Goldberg, J. (1994, January). Helping others through the creative arts. *Career World,* p. 22.

Goodman, R. F. (1992, June 19). Aging artfully: health benefits of art and dance. *Testimony before the U.S. Senate Special Committee on Aging.* Washington, D.C.: U.S. Government Printing Office.

Irwin, E. C. (1984, September/October). The role of the arts in mental health. *Design for Arts in Education, 86,* 43–47.

Kramer, E. (1977). *Art as therapy with children.* New York: Schocken.

Kramer, E. (1979). *Childhood and art therapy: Notes on theory and application.* New York: Schocken.

Kronsky, B. (1986, January). Art therapy through self-exploration. *American Artist, 50,* 12.

Leopold, D. (1997, October). Letter from the editor. *Cyber Journal.*

Lidz, R., & Perrin, L. (Eds.). (1996). Health. *Career information center* (6th ed., Vol. 7, pp. 88–90). New York: Simon & Schuster Macmillan.

Longman, R. (1994, June). Creating art: Your Rx for health. *American Artist, 58,* 68–70.

Lynch, R. T., & Chosa, D. (1996, July/September). Group-oriented community based expressive acts programming for individuals with disabilities. *Journal of Rehabilitation, 62,* 75–81.

McNiff, S. (1986). *Educating the creative arts therapist.* Springfield, IL: Thomas.

Mulder, K. L. (1995, May 15). Hope on the range: B. Voss's art therapy program for troubled youth in San Bernardino County, Calif. *Christianity Today,* p. 59.

Naumburg, M. (1966). *Dynamically oriented art therapy: Its principles and practice.* New York: Grune & Stratton.

Pina, P. (1996, August 31). Psychiatry conference recognises art therapy. *Lancet, 348,* 603.

Pratt Institute, Creative Arts Therapy Department. *Programs of graduate and undergraduate studies, 1998.* Brooklyn, NY: Author.

Rothenberg, E. D. (1994). Bereavement interventions with vulnerable populations. *Social Work with Groups, 17*(3), 61–75.

Samuels, M., & Lane, M. R. (1998). *Creative healing*. San Francisco: Harper.

Schut, H. A. W. (1996, May). Cross modality grief therapy. *Journal of Clinical Psychology, 51,* 357–365.

Ulman, E., & Dachinger, P. (1975). *Art therapy in theory and practice*. New York: Schocken.

Ulman, E., & Dachinger, P. (1996). *Art therapy in theory and practice* (2nd ed.). Chicago: Magnolia Street Publishers.

Ulman, E., Kramer, E., & Kwiatkowska, H. (1978). *Art theory in the United States*. Burlington, VT: Art Therapy Publications.

Ulman, E., & Levy, C. (Eds.). (1980). *Art theory viewpoints*. New York: Schocken.

U.S. Department of Labor. (1991). *Dictionary of occupational titles* (4th ed., Vol. 1). Washington, D.C.: U.S. Government Printing Office.

Wadeson, H.(1987). *The dynamics of art psychotherapy*. New York: Wiley.

Wood, M. M.(1996). *Developmental therapy—developmental teaching: Fostering social-emotional competence in troubled children and youth* (3rd ed.). Austin, TX: PRO-ED.

Zwerling, I. (1992, June 19). Aging artfully: health benefits of art and dance. *Testimony before the U.S. Senate Special Committee on Aging*. Washington, D.C.: U.S. Government Printing Office.

CAREERS IN DANCE/ MOVEMENT THERAPY

WHAT IS DANCE/MOVEMENT THERAPY?

According to a recent publication of the American Dance Therapy Association (ADTA), "Dance/Movement Therapy is the psychotherapeutic use of movement as a process which furthers the emotional, cognitive and physical integration of the individual." It is a nonverbal, action-oriented method of helping people become aware of their feelings by experiencing the sensation of movement. In this case, the human body and its posture, movement, rhythm, and energy serve as the means of communicating the psychological state of the client to the professional. This approach often substitutes for the more traditional method of verbal communication during therapy. It is based on the idea that all thoughts, actions, memories, fantasies, and images involve some muscular tension and that expressive behavior is the motor manifestation of the emotions. Thus, this type of therapy can be effective even with people who have very strong verbal defenses, because the movement can allow for a more reliable expression of feeling than words.

Dance/movement therapy is broadly based on three general assumptions: movement reflects personal traits and abilities, the relationship between the professional and the client enables behavioral change through movement, and changes on the movement level can affect total functioning. The dance/movement therapist is able to assess movement characteristics and overall functioning to determine the client's movement capabilities and style. As with the other expressive therapies, dance/movement therapy serves as both a diagnostic tool and a therapeutic technique to assess dysfunction, as well as to help the client work through emotional and physical blocks, develop greater self-awareness, and increase self-esteem.

Often, the dance/movement therapist works in conjunction with a music therapist for the purpose of stimulating individuals on different sensory levels. However, as with the other creative arts therapies, the aesthetic dimension is far less important than the clients' ability to follow the lead of the therapist, become aware of their own movements, experience improved coordination, and even, at times, be able to improvise movements in response to the music and the emotions.

WHY CHOOSE DANCE/MOVEMENT THERAPY?

A career in dance/movement therapy offers a unique opportunity to combine the desire to help individuals to improve their mental and physical well-being with the desire to develop as a creative or performing artist. One is able to develop and maintain skills in both areas and progress further to assume supervisory and administrative duties and/or enter into private practice. Each option provides the potential for greater professional recognition as well as income.

The increase in the survival rates of critically ill clients as a result of advances in medical technology, as well as the early discharge of clients from hospitals because of managed care policies, have added to the growing need for all kinds of creative therapists. With the increasing proportion of aging adults and the ever-present concern for physical fitness and well-being, the role of the dance/movement therapist will become more significant throughout the human services field. This has been reinforced by the establishment of a Special Committee on Aging of the U.S. Senate and the resulting hearings on the health benefits of art and dance as an aid to effective aging. The variety of settings in which the dance/movement therapist can work, as well as the opportunities for part-time and full-time employment, will further enhance the recognition of this profession.

Obviously, the dance/movement therapist works in close physical contact with many different groups of clients, and the work itself involves a good deal of physical activity. Thus, the essential skills are a strong desire to help others, a full repertoire of interpersonal abilities and physical strength, stamina, flexibility, and coordination. Many dance/movement therapists talk freely of the great sense of satisfaction and accomplishment they experience as professional therapists. An additional advantage, noted by many dance/movement therapists, is the opportunity to stay physically fit as part of their normal working routine.

DEVELOPMENT OF DANCE/MOVEMENT THERAPY—CAREER TRENDS

Dance can be traced back to ancient times. Throughout history, people have expressed themselves through dances of celebration, hope, death, war, and love. It is a commonly held belief that the development of dance therapy in the United States is a result of the dramatic changes that have taken place in the dance form itself. Dance became a creative means for communicating the inner self and a direct outlet for the expression of emotion. This radical shift in dance from the highly structured to the more spontaneous and expressive has served to lay the groundwork for the development of the field of dance/movement therapy.

Almost all of the major pioneers in the field of dance/movement therapy were initially modern dancers who recognized the potential benefits of using dance and movement as a form of therapy. In the late nineteenth century, individuals researched and organized a system of naturally expressive gestures for actors and singers and felt that these gestures could be used to interpret the expressive movements of behavior.

For example, Laban movement analysis (LMA) is based on the premise that movement carries meaning. It recognizes nonverbal experience as something that can be observed, documented, preserved, and analyzed to provide a vocabulary of movement expression as a psychophysical process. The application of LMA to therapeutic intervention and the analysis of interaction patterns and social behavior has been helped by this systematic vocabulary of movement description and interpretation.

The development of dance/movement therapy really was a merging of the essential elements of the development of psychotherapy and modern dance. Traditional psychotherapeutic treatment approaches were usually entirely verbal and nonactive in nature. Similarly, formal dance, as a performing art, also reflected a highly structured, traditional approach. The first half of the twentieth century saw the development of modern dance with a more natural, expressive style of movement emphasizing spontaneity and creativity. At about the same time, psychotherapy was exploring the nonverbal and expressive aspects of personality. Both fields were brought together in the 1940s and 1950s.

When dance therapy began to be acknowledged in the 1940s, its practice was limited to the back wards of mental hospitals. However, by the 1950s, some private practitioners began to apply these techniques to less severely disturbed clients, stressing the development of one's own expressive style based on spontaneity and improvisation. As dance therapy continued to develop during the 1960s, it was still without standardized requirements for professional training and there were very few actual opportunities for training, other than through apprenticeships.

With the establishment of the ADTA in 1966, movement toward a recognized and organized profession began. The development of undergraduate and then graduate coursework in dance therapy took place, and in 1971 the first formal master's degree program in dance therapy was started at Hunter

College in New York City, funded by a grant from the National Institute of Mental Health. Also by that time, the first ADTA Registry Committee was formed to establish criteria for determining levels of professional competence, to establish the ADTA as a professional organization, and to validate dance therapists' professional identity.

Dance/movement therapy plays a significant role in the development of modern institutional human services, such as nursing homes, and in enlivening all long-term care environments. In the 1990s, activities associated with the passive "waiting to die" atmosphere of the older-style institutions are being replaced by more active, participatory, stimulating, creative, and interactive experiences.

What Does the Dance/Movement Therapist Do?

The dance/movement therapist most commonly functions as a member of a therapeutic treatment team, which might include a psychiatrist, psychologist, and social worker. Various other mental health specialists could be added to this team as dictated by the needs of the client, availability of resources, and personnel. Dance/movement therapists can work privately with an individual or with a group.

Dance/movement therapy can be used as a part of an overall treatment plan for an individual or as a primary treatment method. The trained dance/ movement therapist can function as the primary therapist by making interpretations and interventions to help support the emerging aspects of the ego and the self. Because dance/movement therapy sometimes results in a client expressing certain feelings for the first time, the sessions may be part of the diagnosis as well as the treatment.

In some instances, skilled dance and art therapists have combined to develop treatment plans using both forms of therapy. Combined approaches are becoming more common within the expressive therapies field.

Dance/movement therapy can benefit a broad range of people. Therapists work with individuals of all ages who may suffer with social, emotional, and/or physical problems. Dance/movement therapists work with the learning disabled, the visually impaired, the hearing impaired, the autistic, senior citizens, and children. Clients who have been helped by dance/movement therapy also include foster children who have trouble accepting hugs, infants who cannot crawl, fathers who do not know how to play with their children, people suffering from the effects of anorexia and osteoarthritis, and children with attention deficit disorder. Dance/movement therapy has become very popular and useful in treating women with eating disorders, in postsurgical rehabilitation, and as a way of helping pregnant women to feel more at ease with their changing bodies. Of course, the healthy person may also derive great benefits from the expressive qualities of dance/movement therapy. No matter what his or her condition, the individual client undergoing dance/movement therapy does not necessarily have to have a great deal of dance experience or be particularly skilled as a dancer. The ability to move one's body in some form becomes the only necessary prerequisite. Even people who have only limited movement can still be helped.

In work with emotionally disturbed children and adolescents, for example, dance/movement therapy is used to help with problems of low self-esteem, poor body image, poor self-control, lack of trust in others, difficulty in identifying and expressing feelings, and poor interpersonal skills. This helps them develop social competence and express creatively, and nonverbally, their inner anxieties and emotional conflicts in a safe, nonthreatening manner.

Learning disabled individuals with deficits related to receptive and expressive language, reading, writing and mathematics, as well as other areas of disability including motor, attention, memory, perception, self-concept, and social skills, can also be helped. Dance/movement therapy helps these people communicate better, learn to share and cooperate, create, learn new skills, and develop a sense of empowerment and a feeling of success. It often encourages greater risk taking; improves physical strength, mobility, coordination, and flexibility; and focuses on the overall enhancement of the mind-body connection.

In working with hearing-impaired children, the dance/movement therapist must use a vocabulary of signs and gesture, point, and touch in working to convey what is expected and to help clients visualize the rhythm pattern. Using his or her fingers to count visually and beating a drum are two effective ways the therapist can "show" the rhythm to bring about movement.

The use of dance/movement therapy in working with the elderly helps establish communication and carry on a dialogue in movement, which can help break down isolation, promote mental alertness, share feelings, release tension, and improve feelings of independence and self-esteem. It can also encourage reminiscence—the evoking of memories representing the full range of experiences and emotions in a person's life.

One technique used by dance/movement therapists is the formation of a circle. The use of the circle is very important in the work of the dance/movement therapist because it provides the therapist with a visible, physical means of sensing the dynamics of the group and is a way of watching the movement of all the clients, especially the slower ones. The circular formation also helps create a feeling of security and unity. Activities are designed to encourage coordination, concentration, team effort, and timing, as well as exploring interpersonal feelings and establishing personal space.

Within the dance/movement therapy session, the therapist often imitates the client's movements to increase that person's self-awareness. The client is provided with feedback about body rhythm, posture, alignment, expenditure of energy on specific movements, and breathing patterns.

Another technique common to dance/movement therapy is using the client's dreams, fantasies, conflicts, and free association images to portray, through movement and/or dance, as living pictures. Gestures and movements may be symbolic of the root and nature of the specific conflict not yet recognized by the client. Often intense feelings of loneliness, anger, and guilt can be too threatening and overwhelming for words. The expressive qualities of dance/movement therapy can allow these feelings to be conveyed nonverbally.

Another technique is called *improvisation*. During this process, the individual allows the body to move spontaneously. Dance/movement therapists believe that the mind can let go of its control over the body and allow previously guarded emotions and feelings to become visible through the body. Once these emotions are expressed, a greater self-understanding can develop. Dance/movement therapists sometimes use transitional objects (props) such as scarfs or balls to add a dimension to each therapeutic setting. In addition, the use of music, sound effects, and rhythm helps vary the volume and intensity of the movement and helps individuals to feel more involved in the activity. Dance/movement therapists also use videotape to record, preserve, and replay activities.

Dance/movement professionals must also take cultural variables into account, especially in ethnically diverse countries such as the United States. Dance/movement therapists believe that body movement is the most primary means of communication and that techniques can be used to support the individual's struggle toward self-awareness and the connecting of inner psychic processes to the outer world, including the culture in which one exists. In this way, for clients who have great difficulty functioning on a verbal level, the therapist is able to teach and encourage communication and social interactions using nonverbal, culturally symbolic language as a way of expressing thoughts and feelings.

Dance/movement therapy takes place in hospitals, schools, clinics, long-term care facilities, senior citizen centers, adult day care centers, community mental health centers, infant development centers, correctional facilities, and rehabilitation facilities. Therapists also are engaged as consultants and researchers. As the field grows, more dance/movement therapists will be employed in colleges and universities as teachers of dance/movement therapy. In general and psychiatric hospital settings, dance/movement therapists work directly with clients and may also offer training courses to other hospital personnel in the concepts and techniques of dance/movement therapy. A number of dance/movement therapists occupy administrative positions within hospital and institutional settings, such as program directors or supervisors of departments.

Depending on the type of institution and the size of the group, the dance/movement therapist may work in a dance studio equipped with a bar and a wall of mirrors that can be covered by curtains when the mirrors are not in use. The large size of the dance studio permits the group to be divided into smaller groups for certain activities and to permit some degree of free movement when appropriate. Individuals can work with clients in groups or one-on-one.

A Day in the Life of a Dance/Movement Therapist

Gina has been a dance/movement therapist for approximately 12 years in a variety of institutions, mostly hospitals. Having earned bachelor's and master's degrees in physical education, she taught physical education and dance at the collegiate level for many years. Still, she felt that her professional life was lacking the opportunity to truly help people, so she obtained a master's degree in professional studies, with a major in dance/art therapy, which enabled her to qualify for certification as a registered dance therapist (DTR).

Gina then changed her career completely and has worked for the past six years as the only full-time dance/movement therapist at a mental health center affiliated with a large metropolitan hospital. It is a transitional facility providing in- and outpatient services on both a long- and short-term basis. Gina is part of a treatment team consisting of a psychiatrist, psychologist, social worker, psychiatric nurse, and three expressive arts therapists. She has 15 clients whom she sees on an individual basis each week. She also sees these clients in groups once each week.

8:30–9:00 A.M.: Gina meets with the treatment team to review the daily plan for the clients, which may be exercise, walking, relaxation, or daily living skills.

9:00–11:00 A.M.: Gina meets with three clients in individual sessions mostly involving verbal interaction between therapist and client.

11:00 A.M.–Noon: Gina conducts a group dance/movement therapy session with autistic children, and the activity will use the mirrors on the walls to deal with problems related to body image.

Noon–1:00 P.M.: Gina has lunch in the cafeteria and makes some notes about observations she has made of several clients.

1:00–2:00 P.M.: Gina conducts a group session in the large facility with several geriatric clients initially designed to encourage stretching and flexibility. The session progresses to the playing of some European folk dances, which appears to stimulate movement to the rhythm of the music in a group circle and some hand clapping.

2:00–4:00 P.M.: Gina does a substantial amount of paperwork and talking on the telephone dealing with treatment plans, medical reports, lab reports, and assessment of progress, and, increasingly, entering much of this information into a computer.

Each Thursday Gina also attends a lengthy treatment team meeting to discuss those clients who are judged to be in crisis. Information on these clients is exchanged, modification of the treatment is considered, and treatment plans are reviewed and signed by all in attendance. In addition, once every other month Gina participates in case conferences held to discuss all clients, which sometimes includes other consultants.

Gina truly enjoys what she does and has a level of self-confidence that permits her to move easily into therapeutic situations with a sense of optimism and trust in her own abilities. It also helps facilitate her acceptance by other clinical professionals. Although the daily work is strenuous and draining and requires a good deal of flexibility in judgement and spontaneous decision making, she finds it very rejuvenating and personally rewarding.

How Does One Become a Dance/Movement Therapist?

The American Dance Therapy Association is the primary organization charged with the responsibilities for the development and maintenance of all professional standards. The ADTA considers that those entering the field should possess a knowledge of dance; an integration of knowledge and skills generic to dance therapy and practice where emphasis is on utilization of dance movement as the process of intervention; a knowledge of the human body and its functioning; a knowledge of individual and group psychodynamics and process; a systematic approach to movement observation, assessment, and evaluation; experience working with a variety of patient/client populations; an understanding of research design and methodology; and an understanding of one's professional role and responsibility within various settings.

Dance/movement therapists also must be able to work well with other people—clients and other professionals. They must have patience and stamina, a good sense of humor, and a strong desire to help individuals seek positive changes in their lives.

Undergraduate Preparation

Those wishing to pursue a career in dance/movement therapy must first attend an accredited undergraduate academic institution. Currently, a number of undergraduate programs in dance/movement therapy are available. A complete list of schools offering undergraduate and graduate programs in this field can be obtained by writing directly to the ADTA (see "Professional Organizations").

The undergraduate years should be used to gain a broad base of knowledge in related fields, as well as an understanding of dance as an art form. A typical undergraduate program in dance would emphasize courses in the history and philosophy of dance, choreography, dance criticism, survey of dance therapy, dance movement, and classes in ballet, jazz, and modern dance. Courses in biology, anatomy, and physiology are also recommended. Because dance/movement therapists often work with people who have physical problems, an understanding of the physical and mechanical aspects involved in body movement is imperative.

Another element emphasized in undergraduate education is an understanding of human behavior. Because dance/movement therapy is used as a therapeutic tool, developing a broad base of knowledge in psychology is necessary. The student should learn about human personality development, abnormal psychology, group dynamics, and diagnostic testing skills.

Graduate Preparation

According to the ADTA, a master's degree in dance/movement therapy is required for recognition as a professional dance/movement therapist. Therefore, graduate-level education and training will be considered the minimum for an entry-level position. Although most students generally go directly from undergraduate to graduate school, it is becoming more common for a student to gain work experience before entering graduate school. By gaining related work experiences, a student is better equipped to make judgements regarding areas of concentration within graduate school.

Graduate education in dance/movement therapy includes both coursework and internship and requires two years of full-time study. The required coursework usually takes one-and-a-half years and the internship six months. More than half the coursework involves learning specialized techniques that might be applied to various populations. Additional coursework involves developing administrative and research skills. Some students concentrate on developing their clinical diagnostic and evaluative skills, whereas others develop more expertise in learning body movement and body control. Having completed most of the coursework requirements, a student is now ready to use this knowledge as an intern.

Internship is sometimes referred to by other names, such as *fieldwork* or *practicum,* and has the basic goal of providing the student with supervised experience. The dance/movement therapy student is placed in an institution that uses dance as a therapeutic tool and is closely supervised by a graduate faculty member. During this time, the student's skills become refined.

In addition to coursework and fieldwork, dance/movement therapy students are often encouraged to undergo the dance therapeutic process themselves. This will serve to gain additional insights about oneself and understand more fully what the client encounters. Besides formal academic education, a variety of hospital, institute, and agency training programs are becoming more available. These nonacademic programs usually offer specialized training in working with selected populations, such as with autistic children and emotionally disturbed or elderly clients.

LICENSING AND CERTIFICATION

There are two levels of certification for dance/movement therapists. For the first, dance therapist registered (DTR), therapists have received an appropriate master's degree and are fully qualified to work in a professional treatment system. The second, academy of dance therapists registered (ADTR), is for therapists who have met additional requirements and are fully qualified to teach, provide supervision, and engage in private practice after having undergone a number of supervised hours of employment themselves.

The ADTA has also recognized that individuals seeking registration as a DTR may not have access to the most desirable programs in dance/movement therapy as a result of their geographic region. An alternate route is designed for individuals with extensive dance/movement background wishing to pursue master's-level training in dance/movement therapy in combination with study in a related field (that is, social work, psychology, counseling, special education, and dance). For specific information about attaining the alternate route DTR, write to ADTA—Credentials Committee (see "Professional Organizations" for the address).

SALARIES

Salaries in the field of dance/movement therapy vary according to level of responsibility, educational background, experience, and geographic location. For those with proper credentials, starting salaries range from $20,000 to $30,000 per year, those with more experience generally beginning at the upper end of this range. Those individuals who move into the administrative or management responsibilities in an institution may earn between $35,000 and $50,000 per year, with full-time professorial positions in universities potentially earning still more.

A move to administration usually means less direct contact and involvement with clients in the daily activities of the therapy process. Research, teaching, and scholarly writing can enhance one's professional reputation and career and add to income as well.

Dance/movement therapists employed full-time in an institution such as a hospital, school, clinic, or other health care facility usually receive benefits such as health insurance, pension plans, paid holidays and vacations, sick leave, and dental care. Some even provide tuition assistance for further study. Those therapists who are engaged in private practice or who are part-time employees must provide their own benefits.

JOB DESCRIPTIONS

The sample of job descriptions for dance/movement therapists here consists of typical listings obtained from newspapers, journals, and professional newsletters.

Title: Dance therapist

Location: A large mental hospital managed by the Department of Mental Health of an eastern state

Salary range: $23,000 to $26,000 per annum

Qualifications: Minimum of three years' experience working within similar settings. Experience working directly with the more chronically regressed older client. Must be ADTA registered or eligible for registry.

Duties: To work as a member of a therapeutic treatment team with psychiatrist and social worker. To provide direct client care. Some individual and group work with clients will be required.

Title: Dance therapy instructor

Location: Community college on the West Coast

Salary range: $28,000 to $36,000 per annum

Qualifications: Minimum of five years' experience as a practicing dance therapist. Teaching experience mandatory, preferably at the college or university level. Experience teaching history of dance, techniques of dance and movement therapy for emotionally disturbed children. ADTA registered or eligibility for registration.

Duties: To teach introductory and advanced courses in the field of movement therapy and other selected courses as needed with the Department of Physical Education and Health.

Title: Supervisor of Expressive Therapies Department

Location: A large privately funded school for special children in an eastern state

Salary range: $26,000 to $35,000 per annum

Qualifications: Five years of direct client experience plus minimum of three years of experience functioning in a supervisory capacity.

Must have basic knowledge of dance, music, and art therapy, therapeutic techniques. ADTA registered or eligible for registry.
Duties: To direct expressive therapies department and supervise professional staff of five people. Responsibilities include budget preparation, allocation of supplies, and administrative coordination of therapeutic treatment team.

PROFESSIONAL ORGANIZATIONS

American Alliance for Health, Physical Education, Recreation and
   Dance (AAHPERD)
1900 Association Drive
Reston, VA 22091

American Dance Therapy Association
2000 Century Plaza, Suite 108
10632 Little Patuxent Parkway
Columbia, MD 21044-3263
(410) 997-4040

REFERENCES

American Dance Therapy Association. (1996, 1997). [Informational brochures.] Columbia, MD: Author.

Bunney, J. (1992, June 18). Aging artfully: Health benefits of art and dance. *Testimony before United States Senate Special Committee on Aging.* Washington, D.C.: U.S. Government Printing Office.

Burroughs, H., & Kastner, M. (1993). *Alternative healing* (pp. 72–73). La Mesa, CA: Halcyon.

Cole, I. L. (1982). Movement negotiations with an autistic child. *Arts in Psychotherapy, 9,* 49–54.

Creative arts therapists. (1997). *Encyclopedia of careers and vocational guidance* (10th Ed., Vol. 2, pp. 555–560). Chicago: Ferguson.

Freundlich, B. M., Pike, Lynn M., & Schwartz, V. (1989, November/December). Dance and music for children with autism. *Journal of Physical Education, Recreation and Dance, 60,* 50–53.

Groff, E. (1995, February). Laban movement analysis: Charting the ineffable domain of human movement. *Journal of Physical Education, Recreation and Dance, 66,* 27–30.

Hottendorf, D. (1989, November/December). Mainstreaming deaf and hearing children in dance classes. *Journal of Physical Education, Recreation and Dance, 60,* 54–55.

Kleinman, S. (1992, June 18). Aging artfully: Health benefits of art and dance. *Testimony before United States Senate Special Committee on Aging.* Washington, D.C.: U.S. Government Printing Office.

Lappe, M. M. (1984). Dance careers for the next decade. *Journal of Physical Education, Recreation, and Dance, 55,* 76–77.

Lee, S. (1984). Dance administrative opportunities. *Journal of Physical Education, Recreation, and Dance, 55,* 74–75.

Leventhal, M. B. (1993). Moving towards health: Stages of therapeutic unfolding in dance movement. In F. J. Bejjani (Ed.), *Current research in arts medicine* (pp. 257–260). Chicago: MedArt International.

Levy, F. (1988, May/June). The evolution of modern dance therapy. *Journal of Physical Education, Recreation and Dance, 59,* 34–41.

Lowen, A. (1972). *The betrayal of the body.* New York: Collier.

Marr, M. (1975, September). Where do they go when the dancing stops? *Dance Magazine,* pp. 64–65.

Mason, K. (Ed.). (1974). *Focus on dance VII.* Washington, D.C.: American Association for Health, Physical Education, and Recreation.

McNiff, S. (1982). *Educating the creative arts therapist.* Springfield, IL: Thomas.

North, M. (1972). *Personality assessment through movement.* London: MacDonald & Evans.

Pallaro, P. (1993). Culture, self and body-self: Dance/movement therapy across cultures. In F. J. Bejjani (Ed.), *Current research in arts medicine* (pp. 287–291). Chicago: MedArt International.

Sandel, S. L. (1992, June 18). Aging artfully: Health benefits of art and dance. *Testimony before United States Senate Special Committee on Aging.* Washington, D.C.: U.S. Government Printing Office.

Schmitz, N. B. (1989, November/December). Children with learning disabilities and the dance/movement class. *Journal of Physical Education, Recreation and Dance, 60,* 59–61.

Siegel, E. V. (1973). Movement therapy as a psychotherapeutic tool. *Journal of the American Psychoanalytic Association, 21,* 333–343.

Silk, G. (1989, November/December). Creative movement for people who are disabled. *Journal of Physical Education, Recreation and Dance, 60,* 56–58.

Stark, A. (1987, November). American Dance Therapy Association: A kinesthetic approach. *Dance Magazine, 61,* 56–57.

Weeks, S. (1984). *Careers in dance.* Paper presented at Annual Convention of the American Alliance for Health Physical Education and Recreation, Anaheim, CA.

Wislochi, A. (1981). Movement is their medium: Dance/movement methods in special education. *Milieu Therapy, 1*(1), 49–54.

Zalk, K. (1979). Dance therapy. In N. Reynolds (Ed.), *The dance catalog.* New York: Harmony.

ADDITIONAL SOURCES OF INFORMATION

Journals

- *American Journal of Dance Therapy* (Human Sciences Press, 233 Spring St., New York, NY 10013-1578)
- *Journal of Physical Education, Recreation and Dance* (published by AAHPERD)

CAREERS IN MUSIC THERAPY

WHAT IS MUSIC THERAPY?

The American Music Therapy Association (AMTA) defines music therapy as "an allied health profession in which music is used within a therapeutic relationship to address physical, psychological, cognitive, and social needs of individuals." Whether the therapy involves creating music, singing, listening to, or moving to music, it can open up avenues of communication for clients who have limited or no verbal ability, providing an outlet for expressing feelings, motivating people to cope with treatment, and facilitating physical movement and rehabilitation. Because music therapy is essentially nonverbal, it offers a safe and acceptable means of communication for those who need treatment and want to explore therapeutic issues such as self-esteem or personal insight.

Music therapy is one of the components of the general category known as the "expressive therapies" or "creative arts therapies." In this sense it combines the two main disciplines of music and therapy as a therapeutic tool for use in a variety of settings to achieve positive educational, recreational, rehabilitative, preventive, or psychotherapeutic goals. In contrast to other applications of music that may be solely educational or recreational, music therapy encourages communication between client and therapist.

In a therapeutic setting the clinical importance and helpfulness of the music and not its aesthetic or artistic merit are stressed. Aspects of music that may be employed are sound making, rhythm, singing, performing, composing, instrument playing, movement, and coordination or listening. Music is used to engage all the senses, not just the auditory sense, and therefore it is ideal for therapeutic use because so many mental and physical disabilities involve sensory or motor impairment.

Clients who can benefit from music therapy are autistic and emotionally disturbed children, adults with psychotic disorders, individuals who are mentally challenged or learning disabled, inmates, addicts, senior citizens, children with behavior disorders or with a history of abuse, and individuals who experience impaired functioning through speech, hearing, vision, or motor dysfunction. Even individuals considered healthy can improve their lives by applying music therapy techniques for stress reduction, childbirth, pain management, and creative expression.

WHY CHOOSE MUSIC THERAPY?

A career in music therapy offers challenge, opportunities for advancement, and emotional rewards that accompany helping people. As new and innovative uses of music therapy are developed, the music therapist will likely grow along with the field. General and psychiatric hospitals, institutions, agencies, and schools are the most common settings in which music therapists can be found, but positions might also be found in other settings, particularly in schools for children with learning disabilities.

The profession of music therapist, as with some other creative arts therapies, provides an excellent opportunity, with occupational stability, for someone who has a genuine interest in helping people to empower themselves. For individuals who have a background and love of music, who are creative, empathic, patient, imaginative, and open to new ideas and understanding of themselves, the profession can offer a high degree of satisfaction and a chance to make music during the workday and not just during leisure time.

The music therapy profession is growing very rapidly. With the development of the U.S. health care system, forms of expressive therapy are now recognized as being helpful in treating illness of all kinds, and the profession's prestige is growing accordingly. Furthermore, the music therapist is able to exercise independence in developing therapy plans, coordinate with other professionals, and, if desired, engage in private practice as well. Sometimes when full-time positions are not available, qualified therapists contract for part-time work at several institutions. Job opportunities should continue to grow in facilities serving the elderly. Managed care facilities, chronic pain facilities, and cancer care facilities are also hiring more creative arts therapists.

According to the Career Information Center, the employment outlook for music therapists through the year 2005 is very good, with the best chances of employment for those who are prepared to move to geographic areas of greatest demand—in or near large metropolitan areas. Job opportunities and salary ranges for certified music therapists vary from state to state.

DEVELOPMENT OF MUSIC THERAPY—CAREER TRENDS

The utilization of music as therapy is almost as old as music itself. Since before recorded history, music has been employed therapeutically to treat the sick using drum rhythms and chanting. Music has been used to reduce pain, treat infertility, achieve altered states of consciousness, and relieve the stress of childbirth. Healing was considered the responsibility of the entire tribe, and music played an important role in helping the individual move from a state of reality to a more spiritualistic level as part of the process. Some of the first written accounts of the influence of music on the human body were mentioned in ancient Egyptian medical records dating back to 1500 B.C. The value of music as a therapeutic aid was recognized by the Pythagoreans in the seventh and sixth centuries B.C. and by Plato in the fourth century B.C. Aristotle observed that music had a cathartic effect on individuals functioning on an emotional level. During the first century A.D., Aristides Quintilianus distinguished between the applications of music to deal with different personality illnesses—one passively listening and the other actively making music.

Intrigued by the possible applications of music, modern society began to explore this subject scientifically. In the sixteenth century a physician identified the value of the music produced by the human voice as being helpful in dealing with psychic disturbances. A noted Russian scientist discovered that certain melodies proved most beneficial in inducing sleep. Scientific findings from his research are still used today to help treat insomnia. In the 1800s Franz Mesmer, the father of hypnotism, used music to assist the patient in achieving the hypnotic state.

The twentieth century brought the technology necessary to both record music and to play this recorded music so that it could be easily brought to bear in health care treatment at a variety of facilities.

The profession of music therapist developed fairly rapidly in the United States as a result of the need to address the complex problems presented by returning World War II veterans to many hospitals. These were not only physical problems but mental and psychosocial as well. The positive effects of music as performed and as listened to were quite obvious, but it was also apparent that therapeutic application on deeper levels was needed. As a result, a group of musicians, music educators, and psychiatrists convened at the Menninger Clinic in Topeka, Kansas, which ultimately led to the establishment of the first academic training program in music therapy at Michigan State University in 1944.

In 1950 the National Association for Music Therapy was founded. In 1970 the field created a second association called the American Association for Music Therapy. Together these organizations helped establish standards for the field and develop professional criteria for the training of music therapists. Both national associations granted registration (RMT) or certification (CMT) in fulfillment of their respective requirements to those who graduated from an approved college or university program or from an alternative route approved by the AAMT. In 1983, the Certification Board for Music Therapists, Inc., was established to grant board certification (BC) to those candidates who meet its requirements. In 1989, the AAMT created the status of advanced certification (ACMT).

The American Music Therapy Association was founded in 1998 as a union of the American Association for Music Therapy and the National Association for Music Therapy. Its role is to support the therapeutic use of music in hospital, educational, and community settings and to lead the profession by setting criteria for academic and clinical training, as well as the professional registration and certification of music therapists. Music was the first of the creative arts therapies to offer university-level training in the United States, and many colleges and universities now offer degrees in music therapy. The research in music therapy has tended to focus on specific problems such as autism, behavior disorders, and cognitive disorders and to have much more of a scientific basis than the other creative arts therapies.

The development of managed health care systems has become increasingly more important as the number of creative arts therapists has grown in institutionalized settings. Their effect on how the institutions and individual practitioners make decisions regarding the services provided, the length and degree of treatment, and the amount of freedom and autonomy on the job will be significant in the years ahead.

WHAT DOES THE MUSIC THERAPIST DO?

The music therapist most commonly functions as a member of a therapeutic treatment team that often includes physicians, psychologists, psychiatrists, and social workers. Other mental health specialists could be added to this team when dictated by the needs of the specific client and the availability of resources and personnel. The music therapist can work privately with an individual or with a group. The person undergoing music therapy does not necessarily have to possess any musical talent or have prior musical experience.

Whereas the client does not need a high level of musical proficiency, the music therapist certainly does. Most music therapists play several instruments such as the piano, guitar, recorder, flute, or harmonica. In addition, music therapists should be able to sight-read music and play by ear. The development of these skills requires lengthy study and practice. Music therapy can also be thought of as a means of diagnosis as well as therapy, in which the music serves as a replacement for words with clients who have verbal difficulty. After making a diagnosis and determining the severity of the problem, the music therapist assigns the client to either individual or group-oriented music therapy. As a member of the treatment team, the music therapist helps plan activities to meet the needs, abilities, and interests of clients. After working with clients, using varied approaches, the music therapist usually confers once again with the treatment team. The therapist would probably discuss the client's responses to certain activities. Together with the combined advice of this team, the music therapist evaluates the continued needs of the client and plans new activities to help reach the desired goals.

In working with adults, the music therapist uses elements such as long-term memory, abstract thought, and musical preferences that adults have developed. In people with cognitive disorders such as Alzheimer's disease, access to the memory becomes essential in providing treatment. Music that reflects an individual's past often results in emotional reactions, thereby providing an opportunity to reach a client by evoking attention, emotional response, and recognition of the familiar. The music therapist must carefully observe reactions and change the music accordingly to stimulate as well as support any client reactions. The repetition of familiar songs in subsequent music therapy sessions can help promote heightened recognition, enhanced memory recall, and increased eye contact, attention, and self-awareness. Rhythm serves to stimulate attention and promote spontaneous movement, thereby improving muscle flexibility and motion.

Research has found that music has the effect of relaxing the voluntary muscles. As a result, music therapy has been found helpful in the treatment of headaches, insomnia, anxiety, emotional crises, and loss of self-awareness. As part of the relaxation process, music helps facilitate the visualization of positive scenes and images. Music may stimulate the body to produce natural painkillers, or *endorphins,* and thus reduce stress. Noting this effect, many hospitals play music in pre- and postoperative facilities and delivery rooms.

Music-based individualized relaxation training (MBIRT) has been identified as a therapy using one or more elements of music to elicit and/or shape one or more behaviors needed to eventually reach relaxation. MBIRT is presented as an alternative to traditional medication treatment for individuals with cognitive or behavioral deficits such as the elderly, developmentally disabled, and severely disturbed. The objective is to match the musical stimuli to the individual's mood and then to change the mood in the desired direction by changing the musical stimuli. This eventually would have the effect of reducing undesirable behaviors and eliminating the need for medication to control behavior.

In working with learning disabled children, who are unable to understand their senses, who have scattered attention, or who overreact, the arts provide the structure and discipline that help them succeed. In dealing with children, often overlooked are the gains in socialization from musical experiences. Children are aroused by the sounds and rhythms, they become aware of other children, and they remain involved and participating using the instruments. Songs and other vocal sounds stimulate basic language processes. Musical activities can be effectively combined with other activities such as art, so that children have an opportunity to actually express in a visual sense how the music sounds even when they cannot do it verbally. Furthermore, music can provide the background for stories or for drama and dance. Musical groups provide opportunities for children to lead and work together to plan an activity.

Music therapists usually use an assortment of musical instruments: cymbals, finger cymbals, tambourines, drums, triangles, xylophone, and sticks. Clients select instruments and a group leader, or the music therapist leads the group in a particular rhythm. Sometimes clients sit in a circle without instruments and clap their hands and/or stomp their feet to imitate rhythms.

A group may also listen to a prearranged selection of music. The music is often rather abstract in nature, consisting of melodies combined with sounds, such as the ringing of bells, horns, birds chirping, wind, and water. In music therapy with an individual, the client is able to select an instrument and determine what he or she will play in terms of rhythm, tempo, sound, and volume.

In addition to working with clients in groups or individually, the music therapist must often attend meetings with other professional members of the treatment team, write reports about client responses to treatment, select background music, arrange for concerts for or by the clients, accompany or lead singing or rhythm groups, teach music to individuals or groups, encourage musical creativity in the clients, and direct vocal or instrumental groups. In addition to the therapeutic responsibilities, the music therapist usually orders and maintains equipment and supplies such as instruments, electronic equipment, tapes, and sheet music. Another important part of the music therapist's job is to educate others about the field, such as other professionals and the general public.

Music therapists work in a variety of both public and private settings. The most common and more traditional are general and psychiatric hospitals, schools, community mental health centers, retirement homes, settlement houses, day care centers, learning disabled centers, substance abuse treatment centers, rehabilitation centers, hospices, oncology treatment centers, pain/stress management clinics, and special services agencies. A number of nontraditional programs using the skills of music therapists are being created in correctional facilities for both youths and adults. In addition, many business firms are employing music therapists as consultants to design music environments for their employees. Personal growth centers are employing music therapists to work with a traditional population to achieve greater self-expression and self-understanding.

As the field continues to grow, more music therapists will begin to occupy positions as administrators, supervisors, and directors of programs. An increasing number of music therapists are actively engaged in conducting research projects in clinical, educational, and rehabilitative settings. In colleges and universities, many music therapists are involved directly with teaching responsibilities within music therapy programs. As the scientific research conducted in the field increases, it may create additional employment opportunities for trained music therapists in a variety of innovative settings. Also, music therapists provide consultative services to other music educators and special educators in their direct service to students with disabilities.

Music therapy can even take place in the home, particularly in dealing with individuals such as older adults who are homebound. A home-based program where participants can learn music-listening, stress-reducing techniques through weekly home visits by a music therapist may help reduce feelings of distress and depression, while improving mood and self-esteem.

A Day in the Life of a Music Therapist

Steve is employed as a full-time music therapist in a psychiatric unit of a large metropolitan hospital in a big city. This is called an acute unit and consists of adults who remain in the facility for at least two weeks, during which time they are observed and evaluated by a team of professionals to determine the appropriate subsequent treatment at a long-term facility. The patients exhibit symptoms that may be drug related, geriatrically related, and mental as well as medical in nature.

Steve possesses a bachelor's degree in music and a master's degree in music therapy. He has been certified by the National Association for Music Therapy by virtue of his academic preparation and a one-year internship. A typical day for Steve is as follows:

8:30–9:30 A.M.: Steve participates in the morning rounds conducted by a team of professionals consisting of a medical doctor, nurse, social worker, and the activities therapist. The nurse reports on the behavior of the patients during the previous evening, and Steve adds his observations of the patients as they are relating to each other and participating in the group. The team discusses possible recommendations for further treatment, discharge, or changes in treatment.

9:30–10:15 A.M.: Steve meets with his morning group consisting of about 15 patients in a large open room in which he has already set up several musical instruments (usually percussion instruments), surrounded by chairs set in a circle. During this period, Steve provides the leadership for the group by playing the melody on a keyboard or guitar while the patients play the percussion instruments to provide the rhythm component. Steve encourages the patients to dance, move, move their hands, exercise and breathe, as well as to relate to each other and even share in the playing of a drum. Usually there is a theme song for the day, and the patients are encouraged to vocalize when possible and appropriate.

10:15–10:30 A.M.: Steve uses this brief break time to make written notes about the group activity for review later in the day or week.

10:30–11:30 A.M.: Steve conducts individual sessions with those patients deemed to be higher functioning. He encourages individuals to listen to music or create songs with the help of the activities therapist. Usually these sessions last about thirty minutes.

11:30–Noon: Steve continues to make notes on the observations he has made in the group and individual sessions.

1:00–3:00 P.M.: After lunch, the team meeting that began earlier in the day continues with discussion of each of the patients in the group in greater depth. Once or twice a week Steve meets with his supervisor, who is a more experienced activities therapist now acting in an administrative capacity. Participants discuss needed materials and supplies, the facilities being used, and the other resources that may be needed to do their jobs more effectively. In addition, discussion sometimes takes place about the relationship between Steve and the other members of the team and how this can be improved.

3:00–3:15 P.M.: Steve prepares for another group session with the same patients as earlier in the day, but with the idea of planning a different activity such as singing, dancing, drawing to music, or enjoying a social hour with the group members.

3:15–4:30 P.M.: Steve does more paperwork and record keeping, including the assessments of the patients. In addition, he interviews new patients and assesses their level of functioning, grooming, activity, and interest.

4:30 P.M.: The regular work day is over. However, twice each week the schedule is changed to run from noon until 8 P.M. for the purpose of having evening activities such as a movie, relaxation exercises, or listening to music.

Steve very much enjoys his career as a music therapist and feels challenged when that role expands, for it permits him to become more creative, spontaneous, and interdisciplinary in his approach to patients. He feels that he has been adequately prepared for her work through his formal academic training and, most of all, his training through the internship. He wishes he had more time to become involved in his own professional development but is constantly confronting the pressures of limited time, energy, and financial support for this important purpose. He is considering the possibility of becoming a supervisor in the near future and obtaining the necessary training for this.

HOW DOES ONE BECOME A MUSIC THERAPIST?

The aspiring music therapist must possess good physical health for stamina and good emotional health to work with different types of people and to be a good role model. The music therapist should also have a sincere interest in helping people, patience, tact, understanding, the ability to cope with frustration, and a good sense of humor. In addition, the successful music therapist should be a good musician, creative, imaginative, and have good interpersonal skills.

Undergraduate Preparation

To become a professional music therapist, one must first complete a four-year course of study with a major emphasis in music at an AMTA-approved college or university. Today 71 schools offer bachelor's programs specifically in music therapy. The academic preparation and clinical training of the music therapist can be accomplished through different options approved by the AMTA. An individual can complete a baccalaureate degree in music therapy followed by a six-month clinical internship in an approved mental health, special education, or health care facility. Another option, for those who have completed a baccalaureate degree in music, is to complete a degree equivalency program in music therapy at an approved university in which the student completes only the specified additional coursework without the need to complete another bachelor's degree.

The training of a music therapist is multidisciplinary, in that it involves subject areas other than music, although music therapy degrees, compared with the other creative arts therapies, place greater emphasis on artistic development and skills than on clinical development. A student with a major emphasis in music must earn approximately half of all college credits in music courses. A typical program of study includes coursework in music therapy, music arranging, history of music, music conducting, and vocal and instrumental studies. In addition to the coursework in music, a student needs a background in biology, psychology, sociology and general education.

Graduate Preparation

Currently 23 schools offer graduate programs in music therapy. Graduate schools vary in the type of curriculum offered but in general focus on developing skills in specific areas of music therapy such as musical arrangement, conducting, or advanced work with instruments. Master's degree programs expand the discussion on issues, clinical techniques, and research inquiry into the field. In addition, graduate training offers the student the opportunity to develop more skills and gain additional background in working with different populations. Positions as supervisors or directors of music therapy programs will likely be filled by those who hold advanced degrees.

At this point, there is no AMTA-approved doctoral degree program in music therapy, although some university doctoral programs offer coursework in music therapy as part of the study of a related academic discipline. If the field develops at its present pace, however, it may not be long before doctoral-level programs in music therapy will be available throughout the country.

LICENSING AND CERTIFICATION

To become recognized as a professional music therapist, one must be accepted for certification with the AMTA. State or government agencies do not certify music therapists; it is the responsibility of the AMTA to do this. Certification by the association follows college graduation and completion of an approved internship. Upon successful completion of the undergraduate and clinical training, the student is then eligible to take the certification examination administered by the Certification Board for Music Therapists, Inc. This procedure ensures that the music therapist has at least completed the minimum criteria established for professional competence. Most institutions, agencies, and schools require the music therapist be certified. A list of criteria for training and certification procedures is available from the AMTA (see "Professional Organizations").

For those music therapists who want to work within public school settings, a separate teaching license is often required. Criteria for teaching licenses vary from state to state. Normally a person can fulfill teaching license requirements by completing various teacher training courses as part of the undergraduate program. To obtain a list of criteria needed for teacher licensing, one can write directly to the state department of education.

SALARIES

Earnings vary by the type of institution in which one is employed, the title of one's job, the amount and type of previous experience, the level of educational and clinical preparation, and the geographic area. In general, though, beginning salaries for music therapists are between $19,000 and $25,000 per year depending on the nature of the institution and the part of the country. Music therapists with a master's degree will most likely earn more, with average salaries between $25,600 and $33,500 per year. Those who possess a doctoral degree and teach in a university setting can earn $50,000 or more per year. Professionals who are engaged in private practice can earn substantially more as a supplement.

Full-time music therapists usually receive an array of fringe benefits such as health insurance, pension plans, paid holidays and leaves, dental benefits, life insurance, and, in some cases, tuition assistance for further study. The majority of music therapists are employed in institutions and for the most part work 40 hours per week. In these settings, advancement and increased income generally occur as a result of movement to supervisory or administrative positions, thereby leaving clinical practice.

JOB DESCRIPTIONS

The following represent a selected sample of job descriptions for music therapists based on typical listings obtained from newspapers, journals, and professional newsletters.

Title: Full-time music therapist
Location: A California hospital
Salary range: $2,739 to $3,002 per month + benefits
Qualifications: Bachelor's degree in music therapy and completion of approved clinical internship.
Duties: Music therapist will provide therapeutic rehabilitation activities for adult, forensic psychiatric patients. Therapist will serve as the unit activity coordinator, provide inservice training to patients and staff, conduct assessments, formulate treatment objectives and plans, work with interdisciplinary team, and document patient progress. Therapist may work with volunteers and student interns.

Title: Full-time music therapist
Location: Maximum-security forensic inpatient program in the Midwest
Salary range: $1,754 to $2,605 monthly
Qualifications: Bachelor's degree in music therapy, MT-BC.
Duties: Position available to provide music therapy services to psychiatric adult and geriatric patients. Will provide group and individual music therapy sessions in a psychosocial rehabilitation program. Excellent benefits including retirement, health, fifteen days' annual leave, ten days' sick leave, twelve holidays, life insurance, and more.

Title: Full-time music therapist
Location: New York State
Salary range: $22,000 to $24,000
Qualifications: Bachelor's degree in music therapy; board certification preferred.
Job duties: Provide large- and small-group music therapy services to children ages two to twenty-one with multiple disabilities.

Title: Full-time music faculty at an urban university
Salary range: $30,823 to $77,829 for the academic year; summer teaching may be available.
Qualifications: Master's degree in music therapy; MT-BC; minimum of three years of successful music therapy clinical experience beyond the internship; faculty authorization from NAMT or AAMT; strong background in guitar. Doctorate, university-level teaching, and expertise in applied low strings or double reeds are preferred. Successful performance in an on-campus interview, including a teaching session, is required. Perceived ability to work productively with students and colleagues required. Preference will be given to candidates demonstrating familiarity with a broad range of continuous techniques, the use of instructional technology in the teaching-learning process, and the role of faculty in student success, recruitment, and retention.
Duties: Teaching undergraduate courses in music therapy, supervising music therapy clinical practica, teaching Class Guitar I and Class Guitar II, as well as academic advisement, scholarly activities, related services, and other duties as assigned.

Professional Organizations

American Music Therapy Association, Inc.
8455 Colesville Road, Suite 1000
Silver Spring, MD 20910
(301) 589-3300
www.musictherapy.org

References

AJN Newsline. (1995, July). *American Journal of Nursing, 95,* 65–66.
Alvin, J. (1978). *Music for the autistic child.* London: Oxford University Press.
Balch, B. S. J., & Bathory-Kitsz, D. (1993). Composing a new language. In F. J. Bejjani (Ed.), *Current research in arts medicine* (pp. 417–418). Chicago: MedArt International.

Boxhill, E. H. (1993). Multicultural music therapy: A world music perspective. In F. J. Bejjani (Ed.), *Current research in arts medicine* (pp. 399–401). Chicago: MedArt International.

Bruscia, K. E. (1989). *Defining music therapy.* Spring City, PA: Spring City Books.

Burroughs, H., & Kastner, M. (1993). *Alternative healing* (pp. 163–165). La Mesa, CA: Halcyon.

Creative arts therapists. (1997). *Encyclopedia of careers and vocational guidance* (10th ed., Vol. 2, pp. 555–560). Chicago: Ferguson.

Davis, W. B., Gfeller, K. E., & Thaut, M. H. (1992). *An introduction to music therapy.* Dubuque, IA: Brown.

Dubois, Y., & Corti, H. (1982). Games, music and potential space in psychotic children. *Neuropsychiatrie de l'enfance et de l'adolescence, 30,* 437.

Formann-Radl, I. (1993). Music therapy treatment of psychiatric patients. In F. J. Bejjani (Ed.), *Current research in arts medicine* (pp. 375–378). Chicago: MedArt International.

Green, K. (1993–1994, Winter). You're a what? Music therapist. *Occupational Outlook Quarterly,* pp. 43–45.

Gerardi, R. (1991). *Opportunities in music careers* (pp. 125–127). Lincolnwood, IL: VGM Career Horizons.

Hanser, S. B., & Thompson, L. W. (1994, November). Effects of a music therapy strategy on depressed older adults. *Journal of Gerontology, 49,* 265–269.

Larkin, M. (1985, July). Musical healing. *Health, 17,* 12.

Lidz, R., & Perrin, L. (Eds.). (1996). Health. *Career information center* (6th ed., Vol. 7, pp. 88–90). New York: Simon & Schuster Macmillan.

Marwick, C. (1996, January 24/31). Leaving concert hall for clinic, therapists now test music's "charms." *Journal of the American Medical Association, 275,* 267–268.

McGuire, M. G. (1984, September/October). The music therapist: musician or therapist? *Design for Arts in Education, 86,* 19–23.

McNiff, S. (1986). *Educating the creative arts therapist.* Springfield, IL: Thomas.

Sammon, T. J. (1997, September 10). March music—Healing and music. *Journal of the American Medical Association, 278,* 816.

Saperston, B. M. (1993). Music-based models for altering physiological responses. In F. J. Bejjani (Ed.), *Current research in arts medicine* (pp. 379–381). Chicago: MedArt International.

Schwartz, F. J. (1993). Music and medicine. In F. J. Bejjani (Ed.), *Current research in arts medicine* (pp. 375–378). Chicago: MedArt International.

Scofield, M., & Teich, M. (1987, February). Mind-bending music. *Health, 19,* 69–70.

Tomaino, C. M. (1993). Music and the limbic system: Implications for use of music therapy in work with patients with dementia. In F. J. Bejjani (Ed.), *Current research in arts medicine* (pp. 393–397). Chicago: MedArt International.

Wadeson, H. (1976, January), Combining expressive therapies. *American Journal of Art Therapy,* p. 15.

Wood, M. M. (1996). *Developmental therapy—Developmental teaching: Fostering social-emotional competence in troubled children and youth* (3rd ed.). Austin, TX: PRO-ED.

Yanow-Schwartz, J. (1994, December). Experimenting with the arts in education. *American Artist, 58,* 70–74.

Index